Cannabis Policy: Moving beyond Stalemate

D1533472

Cannabis Policy: Moving beyond Stalemate

Robin Room

Benedikt Fischer

Wayne Hall

Simon Lenton

Peter Reuter

Convenor

Amanda Feilding

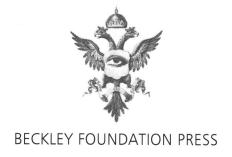

BECKLEY FOUNDATION PRESS

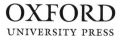

OXFORD
UNIVERSITY PRESS

OXFORD
UNIVERSITY PRESS

Great Clarendon Street, Oxford OX2 6DP

Oxford University Press is a department of the University of Oxford.
It furthers the University's objective of excellence in research, scholarship,
and education by publishing worldwide in

Oxford New York

Auckland   Cape Town Dar es Salaam   Hong Kong   Karachi
Kuala Lumpur Madrid Melbourne Mexico City   Nairobi
New Delhi Shanghai Taipei Toronto
With offices in
Argentina Austria Brazil Chile Czech Republic France Greece
Guatemala Hungary Italy Japan South Korea Poland Portugal
Singapore Switzerland Thailand Turkey Ukraine Vietnam

Oxford is a registered trade mark of Oxford University Press
in the UK and in certain other countries

Published in the United States
by Oxford University Press Inc., New York

The material from this book is a revision of material originally published as the Beckley
Foundation Cannabis Commission Report-Cannabis Policy: Moving Beyond Stalemate, first
launched at the Beckley Foundation Seminar at the House of Lords in October 2008.

ISBN 978-0-19-958148-1

Printed and bound in Great Britain by CPI Antony Rowe,
Chippenham and Eastbourne

Foreword

Calls for reforms in marijuana policy have been a staple of Western discourse for almost 40 years, since the drug first became popular in the late 1960s. I myself was a member of a National Academy of Sciences panel that in 1982 published a report that called for examination of alternatives to the current criminal prohibitions. That report brought an almost unprecedented rebuke from the then president of the Academy who wrote in a Foreword that the committee had gone beyond its competence in raising the issue. The committee most assuredly had not. It was hard to interpret his comment other than as a response to governmental concerns that the issue was an awkward one to raise.

What has indeed been striking has been how little has changed in the ways Western societies deal with a drug whose use has become almost a normal part of the adolescence experience. A few nations and some states in the United States have removed criminal penalties for simple possession of marijuana, but, apart from the Dutch coffee shops, that is almost the limit of experimentation with alternative regimes. In country after country marijuana possession produces large numbers of arrests; in the United States the figure was over 750,000 in 2006 and the per capita rate was comparable in other countries such as Australia and Switzerland. Though very few of these arrests result in sentences of imprisonment, they do represent important intrusions into the lives of many individuals. In the absence of compelling evidence that these arrests reduce marijuana use, it is hard to see the justification for such large numbers.

Many reports have examined the experiences of specific nations with marijuana prohibition. This book is the first that draws on the experiences of a large number of nations. It presents the evidence that marijuana, though capable of causing harm to users, represents a low population health risk and then assesses how policy has been implemented across the Western world, from Australia to Sweden. It is also the first to systematically assess the international regime that underpins the national laws. The authors show the difficulties that the international system presents for any country that wishes to do more than tinker marginally with the existing system.

Another major finding of the book is the failure of legal reform efforts in so many nations to achieve their goals of reducing the intrusiveness of the state. American states that have removed the criminal penalties for possession have kept them for smoking in public, so that arrests have not declined much. In other jurisdictions around the world, removing the criminal penalties for possession has empowered the police to make many more arrests because the paperwork requirements are so much less. It may well be that 'decriminalization' should indeed go further and simply remove all penalties for possession and use; prohibitions on commercial sale might be enough to prevent promotion and thus much expansion of use. The alternative, as the current Governor of California has recommended, is to consider controlled legalization in some form. This study has much to offer those considering either of these paths. It reviews the evidence on what happens down each path, and the ways in which such initiatives and the international regime can be brought into concordance.

For those interested in bringing rationality to marijuana policy, this study is an important work.

Professor Thomas C. Schelling
2005 Nobel Prize Laureate in Economics

Preface

Cannabis is by far the most widely used illegal drug and therefore the mainstay of the 'War on Drugs'. It is used by an estimated 4% of the global adult population, that is, 166 million people out of an estimated population of 200 million illegal drug users'.[1] It therefore constitutes roughly 80% of the 'illegal drug market'. However, cannabis has only ever held a relatively marginal position in international drug policy discussions. In response to its peripheral role in the global debate, I decided to convene a team of the world's leading drug policy analysts to prepare an overview of the latest scientific evidence surrounding cannabis and the policies controlling its use. The report would both bring cannabis to the attention of policy-makers and also provide them with the relevant facts to better inform their future decisions, particularly in the context of the United Nations Strategic Drug Policy Review of 2009, and thereafter.

The historical context of the United Nations' policy is critical here. In 1998, the international community agreed a 10-year programme of activity for the control of illegal drug use and markets. These agreements were made at a United Nations General Assembly Special Session (UNGASS) held in New York in June of that year, and a commitment was made to reassess the situation at the end of the 10-year period. The nature of this programme was epitomized by the slogan 'A drug free world – we can do it!'. However, the reality is that since 1998 drugs have in general become cheaper and more readily available than ever before. We hope that this volume will help lead the way towards a more rational, effective and just approach to the control of cannabis.

Cannabis is, however, a complicated issue, with many seemingly contradictory facets. On the one hand, it has a history of spiritual and medicinal use that dates back millennia; this, together with the explosion in its use during the latter half of the twentieth century, indicates the many subjective benefits that users attribute to it. Moreover, it is one of the least toxic substances used recreationally, where the risk of overdose is negligible. On the other hand, recent years have seen growing concern about an association between cannabis use and a variety of possible harms, particularly mental health disorders.

---

[1] The figures from the UN Office on Drugs and Crime (UNODC) indicate that in 2006–2007 some 166 million people aged 15 or above, or 3.9% of this age group, used cannabis regularly. Just 1% of the world population uses other illegal drugs.

Only through extensive and rigorous research can we hope to clarify the contradictions between the perceived benefits of cannabis and the dangers it presents.

Some of the many questions on which we lack reliable evidence include: Why do people choose to use cannabis? What are the psychological and therapeutic needs it fulfils? What are the processes it might enhance? Why and when is cannabis harmful? Can this be understood in terms of differences in individual genetic and personality types, or in the type of cannabis consumed, or in the pattern of its consumption? By answering these and other questions we might minimize the harms caused by cannabis use and help to prevent its misuse, as well as better understanding the benefits many users reportedly derive from it, both in alleviating sickness and promoting well-being.

When considering harms, it is also important to include the adverse effects of a criminal justice approach to cannabis control. This is particularly pertinent given the evidence that cannabis control policies, whether draconian or liberal, appear to have little or no impact on the prevalence or intensity of its consumption. Indeed, at the onset of international cannabis prohibition, use of the drug was confined to a scattering of countries and cultures, but since then it has spread around the world and is now widely used in most developed countries, to the extent that it has become a rite of passage for a majority of young people.

In the developed world, it is all too easy to overlook the unintended consequences of the War on Drugs, including the extensive violations of human rights, since in these countries the violations are most predominantly felt by drug-users themselves, particularly where discriminatory enforcement leads to significantly higher levels of arrests among the disadvantaged and minority groups. However, in producer/transit countries, such as in Latin America, the suffering caused by this war is vastly more widespread, affecting not only farmers but also whole populations by the destabilization of political and social systems through corruption, violence, and institutional collapse. While attention to these systemic effects has primarily been focused on other drugs, the war on cannabis also plays a significant role.

However, despite cannabis being responsible for the great majority of arrests for illicit drug-use – in the US alone approximately 750,000 arrests per annum – international drug policy discussions have tended to ignore cannabis, focusing instead on those substances that cause the most harms: opioids, cocaine, and amphetamines. As discussed in this volume, although cannabis has always been marginal to the main interests of the international drug control system, the upholders of the system have been extremely reluctant to consider reforms which would change its status within, or remove it from, that system.

Although this Report is specifically targeted at reviewing cannabis laws, it is worth noting that any change to the scheduling of cannabis under the international drug control system could lead to the questioning of the whole War on Drugs approach. Without cannabis within the system's remit, the number of illegal drug-users in the world would total somewhere in the region of 40 million people – arguably too small a number to justify the vast costs, in money, human suffering, and political corruption, of the current efforts to enforce the ideals behind this unwinnable war. With a much narrower target the War on Drugs might turn instead into a more sensible campaign to relieve the problems caused by the dependence of a small number of users on more addictive and dangerous drugs.

The present volume reviews the issues which need to be considered by policy-makers in developing more effective cannabis policies that minimize the harms associated with its use and control. We hope that this Report will prove useful in policy discussions concerning cannabis, not only in the context of the 2009 international review, but also as a guide for governments seeking to reform their cannabis policies thereafter, and that it will further promote a wider discussion of these important issues amongst the general public.

Amanda Feilding
Director of the Beckley Foundation

Acknowledgements

We thank each of the following, who provided help or advice on specific points: Laurence Helfer, Les Iversen, Martin Jelsma, Shekhar Saxena, and Ambros Uchtenhagen. Particular thanks are due to Louisa Degenhardt for graciously allowing us to draw on her collaborative work with Wayne Hall. Wim Scholten and Bob Keizer provided useful advice at a Beckley Foundation meeting on the project. We also thank each of the following, who provided research or information assistance: Jude Gittins, Jonny Hazell, and Katherine Rudzinski; and Sarah Yeates for assistance in locating the literature on the health effects of cannabis and in formatting the chapter on the health effects of cannabis. Thanks also to Maggie Halls for her assistance in locating reference material for chapters on the range of reforms and their effects.

While the Beckley Foundation provided the major support for this project, each author's work on this book was also part of their broader program of research and scholarship supported by a variety of public funding bodies and private foundations. We acknowledge the support both of these bodies and of the research centres and universities which are our primary employers. The Beckley foundation would also like to give special thanks to the public and private foundations that have supported this work, including the J. Paul Getty Jr. Charitable Trust and the San Francisco Foundation.

The authors would like to give special thanks and appreciation to Amanda Feilding, Lady Neidpath, the founder and director of the Beckley Foundation and our convenor. The report on which this book is based was Amanda's idea in the first place, and she has been instrumental in bringing it into being, patient and helpful with suggestions, and gracious and hospitable throughout the process.

Contents

Part I

Cannabis Policy: Moving beyond Stalemate

Chapter 1

Introduction

Cannabis as an issue

Marijuana is the most widely used illegal drug in the world. The United Nations Office of Drugs and Crime (UNODC) estimates that, across all nations, 160 million people used cannabis in the course of 2005, 4% of the global adult population – far more than the number that used any other illicit drug, though far less than the number that consumed alcohol or tobacco. The number of cannabis users in 2005 was 10% higher than estimated global use in the mid 1990s (UNODC, 2007). The numbers are particularly striking because fifty years ago cannabis was a very uncommon drug, with pockets of traditional use in India, Jamaica and a few other developing nations and use otherwise largely confined to fringe bohemian groups in a few rich countries.

All nations prohibit both the production and use of cannabis and have been committed to do so at least since ratifying the 1961 Single Convention on Drugs. The spread of cannabis use among adolescents and young adults led to a strong reaction in much of the developed world, which still results in large rates per capita of arrests for cannabis possession and use in nations such as Switzerland, Australia and the United States. The emergence of a new stream of research findings documenting that cannabis can trigger adverse mental health consequences for some users has recently increased popular concern.

On the other side of the policy debate there is a concern, dating back to the 1970s, that the state is intruding too much into personal life in its efforts to control cannabis use, and that criminal penalties are not justified for an offence that risks harm largely only to the user. There has been a long-term trend toward less punitive policies in such countries as Australia, Great Britain, the Netherlands and France, although actual patterns of policing have often undermined the trend. Now the direction of trends is less clear, in part influenced by new evidence on cannabis and mental disorders.

Using cannabis: who, where, why?

Cannabis, like other psychoactive substances such as alcohol, tobacco and opiates, is used for a variety of reasons. For some users it is simply the pleasure of an altered state and a social experience. For others, it is a way of coping with the troubles of everyday life, a source of solace or, indeed, a source of cognitive benefits and enhanced creativity (Iversen, 2008). For yet other users it has a therapeutic value for some physical or mental health problem. Though the medical value of cannabis is not well researched, it is plausible that it does in fact provide relief for a number of conditions, such as AIDS wasting syndrome or glaucoma (Joy et al., 1999).

Cannabis first became popular in the West in the 1960s, when its use emerged as part of the general youth rebellion of that decade. From North America it spread, over the next twenty years, to most of Western Europe, as well as to Australia. After the collapse of the Soviet Union, it also spread in the 1990s to many countries in Eastern Europe. There is, however, substantial variation in rates of use across these nations: Finland and Sweden, for example, have rates of users on a lifetime basis that are about two-fifths the rate in Great Britain (EMCDDA, 2007: Table GPS-8). In the countries with high rates of cannabis use, roughly half of all adults born since 1960 have used the drug.

Cannabis is now used in every region of the world. The percentage of adults who report use in the past year was higher than the global average in Oceania (16%), North America (11%), Africa (8%) and Western Europe (7%). It was at or below the global average in Eastern Europe (4%), South America (2%), South-East Europe (2%) and Asia (2%) (UNODC, 2007). Because of their larger populations, Asia and Africa accounted for 31% and 24% of global cannabis use respectively, followed by the Americas (24%), Europe (19%) and Oceania (2%).

The United States and Australia have conducted surveys of drug use since the mid-1970s and mid-1980s respectively (AIHW, 2007; SAMHSA, 2006). In the United States in 2005, 40% of the adult population reported trying cannabis at some time in their lives, with 13% of adolescents reporting use in the past year (SAMHSA, 2006). In Australia in 2007, 34% of persons over the age of 15 reported that they had used cannabis at some time in their lives (AIHW, 2008).

Rates are highest among youth, particularly young adults, and use tails off slowly in the mid-30s. At the other end of the age of use spectrum, the age of first use has fallen since about 2000 in some countries, but not others (Hibell et al., 2004; Degenhardt et al., 2000).

Cannabis use in the USA typically begins in the mid to late teens, and is most prevalent in the early 20s (Bachman et al., 1997). Most cannabis use is intermittent and time-limited, with very few users engaging in daily cannabis use over a period of years (Bachman et al., 1997). In the USA and Australia, about 10% of those who ever use cannabis become daily users, and another 20% to

30% use weekly (Hall & Pacula, 2003). Cannabis use declines from the early and mid-20s to the early 30s, reflecting major role transitions in early adulthood (e.g. entering tertiary education, entering full-time employment, marrying, and having children) (Anthony, 2006; Bachman *et al.*, 1997). The largest decreases are seen in cannabis use among males and females after marriage, and especially after childbirth (Bachman *et al.*, 1997; Chen & Kandel, 1995).

While marijuana use, once it is established in a society, seems never to fall to very low rates, there has been substantial variation in prevalence over the last decades. For example, whereas in 1979 50.8% of American high school seniors had used marijuana in the previous twelve months, by 1992 that figure had fallen to 21.9%; it then rose again to 37.8% in 1999 (Johnston *et al.*, 2007). Interestingly, there seems to be a common pattern over time across countries. For most western nations between 1991 and 1998 there was an increase of about half in the proportion of 18 year olds reporting that they had tried cannabis. Since 1998 in the same countries there has been a substantial decline in that figure, though in 2006 it still remained well above the 1991 level.

The common patterns across countries with very different policy approaches reinforce the general impression that penalties for personal use have very little impact on the prevalence of cannabis use in a society. What does explain the changes remains essentially a mystery, but popular youth culture, including representation of the drug in music, films and magazines, probably plays an important role. The linked patterns of fluctuation in use in different countries suggest the influence across borders of a global youth popular culture.

Marijuana use can be thought of as a 'career'. Most users try the drug a few times, and are at very low risk of suffering or causing any substantial harm. However recent research has confirmed that a substantial fraction will use the drug regularly over the course of ten or more years, and that perhaps 10% of those trying cannabis at some stage will become dependent upon it. Among those who begin to use in their early teens, the risk of developing problem use may be as high as one in six (Anthony, 2006). It is worth comparing the drug's use in these respects to alcohol and tobacco on the one hand, and to cocaine and heroin on the other. Cannabis is most like alcohol, in that most users do not become dependent but many do have using careers that stretch over years, although in current circumstances not for as long as for alcohol.

Forms of cannabis: the plant and the preparations

Cannabis preparations are primarily derived from the female plant of *Cannabis sativa*. The plant contains dozens of different cannabinoids (ElSohly, 2002; Iversen, 2007), but the primary psychoactive constituent in cannabis products is delta-9-tetrahydrocannabinol (THC) (Iversen, 2007; Pertwee, 2008). Administration of THC in pure form produces psychological and physical effects that are similar to those users report when they are smoking cannabis (Wachtel *et al.*, 2002), and drugs that block the effects of THC on brain receptors also block the effects of cannabis in animals (Pertwee, 2008) and humans (Heustis *et al.*, 2001). The effects of THC may also be modulated by cannabidiol (CBD), a nonpsychoactive compound that is found in varying amounts in most cannabis products (Iversen, 2007).

The THC content is at its highest in the flowering tops of the female cannabis plant. Marijuana (THC content in the range of 0.5% to 5%) comprises the dried flowering tops and leaves of the plant. Hashish (THC content in the range of 2% to 20%) consists of dried cannabis resin and the compressed flowers. Hash oil is an oil-based extract of hashish that contains between 15% and 50% THC (UNODC, 2006). Some varieties of marijuana such as Sinsemilla (skunk) and 'Nederwiet' ('Netherweed') may have THC content as high as 20% (EMCDDA, 2006).

Cannabis is usually smoked in a 'joint', the size of a cigarette, or in a water pipe, with tobacco sometimes added to assist with burning. A typical joint contains between 0.25 and 0.75g of cannabis. The amount of THC delivered to the lungs varies between 20% and 70%, and 5% to 24% reaches the brain (Hall & Solowij, 1998; Heustis, 2005; Iversen, 2007). A dose of around 2 to 3 mg of bioavailable THC will produce a 'high' in occasional users, who usually share a joint between multiple users. More regular users can use three to five joints of highly potent cannabis a day (Hall *et al.*, 2001). Smokers typically inhale deeply and 'hold' their breath to maximise absorption of THC. Marijuana and hashish may also be eaten, mixed in cakes or cookies (Wikipedia, 2008), or drunk in a liquid infusion (e.g. *bhang lassi* in India), but cannabis is most often smoked because this is the most efficient way to achieve the desired psychoactive effects (Iversen, 2007).

Because of uncertainties about the THC content of cannabis, 'heavy' cannabis use is often defined as daily or near daily use (Hall & Pacula, 2003). Regular use over a period of years increases users' risks of experiencing adverse health and psychological effects (Hall & Pacula, 2003). Daily cannabis users are more likely to: be male, be less well educated, and regularly use alcohol, tobacco, amphetamines, hallucinogens, psychostimulants, sedatives and opioids (Hall & Pacula, 2003).

Prohibiting a plant that grows almost anywhere

Prohibition may reduce cannabis use by making the drug more expensive and harder to get. We review the evidence on this in Chapter 3. It may also shorten use careers. It is also clear that cannabis prohibition has adverse consequences for society by creating large-scale black markets and preventing the effective regulation of a product which can come in forms of varying potency and possibly dangerousness. Though cannabis markets generate less violence than the markets for other prohibited drugs (why is not clear, and would be worth researching), they do generate some tens of billions of dollars in revenues to criminals, and at least modest levels of corruption in some countries. The active enforcement of the prohibitions also leads to very large numbers of arrests and other penalties, each of which can cause considerable harm to the individual beyond any formal sanction that may be imposed, and which are often applied in a discriminatory manner. It is a concern about the disproportionality of these social harms relative to the dangers of the drug itself that is at the heart of many efforts to reform current policies.

Cannabis can be grown almost anywhere, given that it is also very suitable for indoor cultivation. While cocaine and heroin are produced in poor countries and constitute an important source of income for a few source countries, cannabis is produced in many countries, rich and poor, primarily for domestic consumption. The international trade is a much smaller component of the cannabis market than it is for heroin and cocaine.

Cannabis in the international prohibition regime

Almost all countries are signatories to the 1961 and 1988 drug control Conventions, and are required under these conventions to criminalize production, distribution, use or possession of cannabis. Cannabis was brought into the emerging international drug control system in 1925, at the instance of the Egyptian delegate to the Second Opium Conference, but only with respect to medical preparations from the resin (Bruun *et al.*, 1975:183). Cannabis preparations had had wide medical use at the end of the 19th century (Fankhauser, 2008), and in 1952 1000 kg. per year was still used for this purpose (Bruun *et al.*, 1975: 201). Primarily under urging from the US (Bruun *et al.*, 1975: 195–203; Edwards, 2005:153), cannabis was included in the strictest prohibition regime category in the 1961 Single Convention on Narcotic Drugs. This decision was premised on a conclusion that cannabis had no medical value; it was agreed that in the new treaty 'it should … be made clear that the use of cannabis should be prohibited for all purposes medical and nonmedical alike' (10th Session of the CND, quoted in Bruun *et al.*, 1975:199). The fundamental decisions on the status of cannabis in the international regime were thus taken prior to the much wider modern experience with its nonmedical use. The effect of the 1961 Convention was broadened by the provision in the

1988 Convention requiring the production, distribution, possession or purchase of cannabis to be treated 'as criminal offenses under [each country's] domestic law'.

The organs of the international regime

There are three main international bodies with responsibility under the drug control conventions (Room & Paglia, 1999). The Commission on Narcotic Drugs, with 53 nations elected as members by the Economic and Social Council (ECOSOC) of the United Nations, meets annually as the policy-making body. The International Narcotics Control Board (INCB), composed of 13 persons chosen as experts, has a dual role as the manager of the international supply of plant-derived medicines, particularly opiates, and as the watch-dog of the prohibition system for drugs covered by the treaties. The UN Office on Drugs and Crime serves as the secretariat for the system, with a broad international program of work. A fourth international body, the World Health Organization, also has a technical role in evaluating drugs and recommending on how they should be classified under the system.

The place of cannabis in the system

Cannabis is by far the most commonly used substance subject to the system's prohibitions, but it has never been central to the concerns and activities of the system. The discussions of production and trafficking of cannabis in the UNODC's *World Drug Report* 2000, for instance, lacked the specificity of the discussions of opium and coca trafficking. 'Available cultivation and production estimates are not sufficient to determine whether production at the global level has increased or decreased in recent years', the Report remarks (UNODC, 2000:32). The Report went on to note that cannabis seizures rose in the early 1990s, but 'have not increased since the mid-1990s', but added that it is difficult to judge if this reflects 'a real stabilization in global production and trafficking' or shifts in law enforcement priorities. By 2008, a substantial effort had been made to make the global picture for cannabis more concrete. Discussion of the global cannabis situation occupied about one-fifth of the space devoted to specific drug classes (UNODC, 2008:37–169). But this allocation might be compared with the Report's estimate that 65% of global seizures, and 67% of the 'doses' of drugs seized, were of cannabis, and that the estimated global rates of drug use were 3.9% for cannabis, 0.6% for amphetamines, 0.4% for cocaine, and 0.4% for opiates (UNODC, 2008:26, 31).

Indications can be found in all parts of the system of the marginality of cannabis in the system's concerns, at least until recently. The *Bulletin on Narcotics* is a research journal published by the UNODC and its predecessors since 1949 (http://www.unodc.org/unodc/data-and-analysis/bulletin/index. html). Of the 192 articles published in the journal between 1986 and 2006 (the date of the most recent issue), only 10 were on cannabis, 7 of which were in an issue devoted to cannabis in 1994, and one of which was a monograph published in 2008 reviewing the 'world cannabis situation' which is listed as the *Bulletin*'s entire output for 2006 (Leggett, 2008). At its annual sessions, the Commission on Narcotic Drugs passes a series of resolutions, often after heated debate in drafting committees (Room, 2005), and also recommends resolutions to be passed by ECOSOC. Of the 132 CND resolutions passed in the period 1997–2008 (http://www.unodc.org/unodc/commissions/CND/07-reports.html), 4 concerned cannabis (3 of them in 2008); of the 51 resolutions recommended to the ECOSOC, one concerned cannabis. A reading of the annual report for 2007 of the International Narcotics Control Board (INCB, 2008) conveys, on the one hand, the ubiquity of cannabis growing and trafficking as the Board reports on the situation region by region, and, on the other hand, the marginality of cannabis to the system's central concerns. Thus none of the report's 48 recommendations is specifically concerned with cannabis.

At the rhetorical level, however, cannabis has lately come to play an important role in the international drug control regime. The annual statements of the UNODC always mention the estimated share of the world population that use illegal drugs. That number is dominated by cannabis. For example, in the 2005 *World Drug Report* the UNODC stated that there were 200 million drug users globally; of these 160 million (80%) used cannabis. The other drugs listed (ATS, cocaine and opiates) had user populations totaling only 40 million, less than 1% of the world's population. Without cannabis, the totals would suggest that illegal drug use is not a global population-level issue. Thus the drug helps give breadth to the drug issue globally; the same is true in many member nations.

The international system and national and local laws

In its self-conscious role as the 'guardian of the conventions' (Bewley-Taylor & Trace, 2006), the INCB periodically mounts the ramparts on cannabis in defense of the system, for instance by issuing an admonitory press release (UNIS, 2008) in response to press reports of experiments with computerized vending machines by California dispensaries for medical cannabis to be used in accordance with a doctor's letter. A prominent feature of the international drug control system, in fact, is the extensiveness and detail of its concerns with domestic matters in nations which are parties to the treaties.

The level of control over domestic decisions to which the system aspires exceeds, for instance, the level of ambition of the European Union to control national arrangements in the same areas (e.g. concerning the Dutch 'coffee shops' for cannabis), or the power of national governments in federal states to control state or provincial matters (e.g. concerning medical marijuana availability in California and other US states).

In addition to mandating controls on markets in psychoactive substances, the conventions require criminalization of the drug user, if and when the user is in possession of substances that have not been legally obtained. This is an unusually strong requirement even in the context of national laws on contraband commodities, let alone as a requirement of parties to an international treaty; there was no such provision, for instance, in the US alcohol Prohibition laws. The 1961 Convention includes specific provisions that possession of cannabis and other substances controlled by the Convention without legal authority shall not be permitted, and that, where constitutionally allowed, it shall be a punishable offence. As has been mentioned, the 1988 Convention adds the requirement that possession must be made a criminal offence.

A system in stalemate: the system and dronabinol

As noted, the World Health Organization (WHO) plays a technical role under both the 1961 and 1971 Conventions in recommending whether particular substances should be scheduled under either of the conventions, and in which Schedule of the conventions they should be placed. These recommendations are made by an Expert Committee on Drug Dependence, which is now reconstituted for a meeting every two years.

However, the international control system is increasingly inclined to disregard the scientific advice it receives from the WHO. Perhaps the most dramatic instance of this is the turning back by the CND in 2007 of a recommendation for a rescheduling of dronabinol (Δ-9 tetrahydrocannabinol, THC), the principal psychoactive constituent of cannabis, under the 1971 Convention on Psychoactive Substances. Dronabinol is prescribed particularly in the USA under the brand name Marinol as an appetite stimulant, primarily for AIDS and chemotherapy patients. While the plant cannabis and its natural products are included in the 1961 Convention among the substances which are considered the most dangerous and without any therapeutic usefulness (Schedules I & IV), dronabinol was listed under Schedule I of the 1971 Convention (the most restrictive schedule) at the time of that Convention's adoption. The 1989 WHO Expert Committee on Drug Dependence recommended that dronabinol be transferred to Schedule II of the 1971 Convention. The CND initially rejected this, but after a reconsideration by the next Expert Committee made the same recommendation, the CND assented in 1991 (IDPC, 2007).

The 2002 WHO Expert Committee made another critical review, and partly in view of the increased medical use of dronabinol, recommended its reclassification to Schedule IV, the least restrictive schedule. The Executive Director of the UNODC persuaded the Director-General of WHO not to forward this recommendation, claiming it would 'send a wrong signal and create a tension with the 1961 Convention' (IDPC, 2007). The 2006 WHO Expert Committee reconsidered and updated the review. Hesitating between Schedules III and IV, it finally recommended transfer to Schedule III as a small step forward. In its Report for 2006 and at the 2007 CND plenary, the INCB spoke out against the recommendation, expressing concern 'about the possibility of dronabinol, the active principle of cannabis, being transferred to a schedule with less stringent control' (INCB, 2007). In the 2007 CND debate on this, the US was strongly opposed, and many other countries fell in line. Canada commended the WHO Committee for its 'excellent expert advice', but did not support rescheduling because it 'may send a confusing message with regard to the risks associated with cannabis use' (IDPC, 2007). The recommendation was sent back again for reconsideration by the WHO 'in consultation with the INCB' – although the INCB has no formal role in scheduling under the treaties.

Cannabis prohibition and its alternatives: what a policymaker needs to know

The study on which this book is based was commissioned by The Beckley Foundation to inform debate about cannabis policy in connection with the review of the resolutions taken at the 1998 United Nations General Assembly Special Session (UNGASS). UNGASS 98 committed governments to taking action to substantially reduce drug production and demand, including that of cannabis, within the next ten years. The Commission on Narcotic Drugs hosted an international meeting in 2009 to evaluate what has happened in the decade since. However, the Political Declaration painstakingly negotiated over five months and adopted by consensus at the 'high-level meeting' in March 2009 included no detailed analysis of what had actually occurred and was essentially a commitment to the status quo. Thus, at least in the short run, reconsideration of cannabis policies after a half century of international prohibition is left up to policymakers in individual countries and likeminded groups of countries.

This study summarizes what is known about the extent and patterns of cannabis use across nations and over time. It reviews the research literature on the health effects of marijuana use, as well as the little that is known about the other harms associated with cannabis use, production and distribution under current policies. We describe those policies, distinguishing carefully between law on the books and policy as implemented. We emphasize evaluations of the effects on cannabis use and, more broadly, of various kinds of policy innovations aimed at reducing the penalties for personal use.

We give particular attention to the potential for changes in the international treaties that would give nations more flexibility in their policy responses to cannabis. In the final chapter we offer a framework for making cannabis policy decisions and offer some recommendations for policy at the national level.

Our aim is to bring together the present state of knowledge which would be relevant for discussions and decisions about cannabis policy at diverse levels. At the local, state or provincial levels, the problems arising from global policies must be picked up and managed – and much of the action on policy is here because of the stalemate at national and international levels. The national level is the locus not only of decisions about national policy, but also of decisions on national positions on issues in the international treaty system. At the international level, leadership in global efforts and initiatives is needed. We have structured the book as an effort to answer the following empirical questions that need to be answered for informed policymaking.

- What is the state of knowledge about the existence and extent of various potential harms from cannabis use? How does its profile of risk or dangerousness compare to the profiles of other psychoactive substances, licit and illicit?

- How can the present situation and trends be summarized, after half a century of a full global cannabis prohibition regime? How big is the market? How many use, and with what patterns and problems? How many users are caught and punished, and how many receive treatment? What is the evidence on the effectiveness of the prohibition regime in discouraging use and reducing problems? What role does cannabis play in the international drug control regime?

- What are the alternative ways in which the prohibition regime can be ameliorated, to reduce adverse secondary effects? What are the ways which governments have actually used, particularly in terms of reducing or eliminating punishments for possession or use?

- What is the evidence of the effects of these different cannabis policy reform initiatives, on levels and patterns of use, on problems from use, and in reducing the adverse effects of full prohibition?

◆ What alternatives are there under international law for a country or a group of countries wishing to move away from the full prohibition of the present international regime? What is the feasibility and what are the advantages and disadvantages of the different options?

◆ Lastly, we consider what conclusions and recommendations for cannabis control policy we can draw from our analysis.

Chapter 2

The health and psychological effects of cannabis use

Introduction

Any proposal to change the legal status of cannabis must take into account the health and psychological effects of its use. In modern societies, a finding of adverse effects does not settle the issue of the legal status of a commodity; if it did, alcohol, automobiles and stairways, for instance, would all be prohibited, since use of each of these results in substantial casualties. Instead, the scope and extent of the adverse effects become one of the considerations to be taken into account in the policy decisions. The international drug control treaties, and most national drug control laws, divide different psychoactive substances between different 'schedules', with different levels of control and different penalties for trafficking and use, that are supposed to be matched, among other things, to the drug's potential for adverse consequences.

The health and psychological effects of regular cannabis use are not as well understood as those of alcohol and tobacco, but epidemiological research over the past decade has provided evidence that it can have adverse effects on some users, particularly those who initiate use in adolescence and use more than weekly for years during young adulthood. In the decade since the health effects of cannabis were last reviewed by the WHO (Kalant *et al.*, 1999; WHO Programme on Substance Abuse, 1997), there has been a substantial increase in epidemiological and clinical research on the consequences of cannabis use by adolescents and young adults (see Castle & Murray, 2004; Grotenhermen, 2007; Hall & Pacula, 2003; Kalant, 2004; Roffman & Stephens, 2006 for recent reviews).

This chapter summarizes the most probable adverse health and psychological effects of acute and chronic cannabis use. It focuses on those effects that are of greatest potential public health significance, as indicated by their likelihood of affecting a substantial proportion of cannabis users. The adverse effects considered include: the effects of cannabis use on the risk of motor vehicle crashes, a cannabis dependence syndrome, the effects of cannabis smoking on the respiratory and cardiovascular systems, the effects of regular cannabis use on adolescent psychosocial development and mental health, and the effects of chronic cannabis use on cognitive performance and brain function. Priority is given to evidence from well-controlled human epidemiological studies and clinical and laboratory studies of the effects of acute and chronic cannabis use.

At the end of the chapter we consider the evidence in a comparative framework: what can be said about the relative adverse impact on public health of cannabis use compared to use of other psychoactive substances, licit and illicit? As noted, such a comparative perspective is needed for policy decisions about the legal status of cannabis.

Acute health effects of cannabis

Cannabis produces euphoria and relaxation, alters perception, distorts time, and intensifies ordinary sensory experiences, such as eating, watching films, appreciating nature, and listening to music. Users' short-term memory and attention, motor skills, reaction time and skilled activities are impaired while they are intoxicated (Hall & Pacula, 2003; Iversen, 2007). These effects develop rapidly after smoking cannabis and typically last for 1–2 hours (Iversen, 2007). Their onset is delayed for 1–4 hours after oral use (Iversen, 2007).

Cannabis users typically seek one or more of these effects. But use can also result in unsought and adverse effects. The most common unpleasant effects of acute cannabis use are anxiety and panic reactions (Hall & Pacula, 2003; Kalant, 2004). These may be reported by naive users and they are a common reason for discontinuing use. More experienced users may also report these effects after receiving a much larger than usual dose of THC (Hall & Pacula, 2003). Recent research suggests that another constituent present in varying concentrations in cannabis, cannabidiol (CBD), can moderate the psychotogenic effects of THC (Morgan & Curran, 2008), but it remains to be tested whether cannabis products with lower THC:CBD ratios also produce fewer anxiety and panic reactions.

Delta-9-tetrahydrocannabinol appears to produce its effects by acting on specific cannabinoid (CB_1 and CB_2) receptors on the surfaces of cells (Pertwee, 2008). The CB_1 receptor is widely distributed in brain regions that are involved in cognition, memory, reward, pain perception, and motor coordination (Iversen, 2007; Murray et al., 2007). These receptors also respond to a naturally occurring (or endogenous) cannabinoid ligand, anandamide, which produces similar effects to THC but is less potent and has a shorter duration of action (Pertwee, 2008). Neuroimaging studies of the acute effects of cannabis in humans using positron emission tomography (PET) methods confirm findings in animals that THC increases activity in the frontal and paralimbic regions of the brain and in the cerebellum (Chang & Chronicle, 2007).

Acute toxicity and fatal overdose

The acute toxicity of cannabinoids is very low by comparison with other psychoactive drugs, because they do not depress respiration like the opioids, or have toxic effects on the heart and circulatory system like cocaine and other stimulants (Gable, 2004; Kalant, 2004). There have been two reported human deaths from cannabis poisoning in the world medical literature (Gable, 2004), but it is not clear that THC was responsible for these deaths (Kalant, 2004). The dose of THC required to produce 50% mortality in rodents is extremely high by comparison with other commonly used drugs; the estimated fatal human dose is in the range of 15–70g (Gable, 2004; Iversen, 2007), many times greater than the dose that even heavy users could consume in a day (Gable, 2004).

Cannabis increases heart rate and produces complex changes in blood pressure (Chesher & Hall, 1999). There have been reported deaths from myocardial infarction after cannabis use in young adults (e.g. Bachs & Morland, 2001), but these have been rare and they may have occurred in persons with pre-existing, undiagnosed heart disease (Kalant, 2004; and see below).

Accidental injury

The greatest public health concern about the acute effects of cannabis is that intoxicated drivers may cause motor vehicle crashes (Hall & Pacula, 2003). In laboratory studies, cannabis produces dose-related decrements in cognitive and behavioural performance that may affect driving (Ramaekers et al., 2004; Robbe, 1994). Specifically, it slows reaction time and information processing, and impairs perceptual-motor coordination, motor performance, short-term memory, attention, signal detection, and tracking behaviour (Ramaekers et al., 2004; Solowij, 1998). These effects increase with THC dose, and are larger and more persistent in tasks requiring sustained attention (Solowij, 1998).

Surveys find that drivers who report using cannabis are twice as likely to report being involved in accidents as drivers who do not (e.g. Asbridge et al., 2005; Hingson et al., 1982b). It has been difficult to decide how much of the relationship reflects the effects of cannabis on accident risk, the effects of concurrent alcohol use, and the risk behaviour of heavier cannabis users. One recent study found that the association disappeared after controlling for these factors (Fergusson & Horwood, 2001), while another (Blows et al., 2005) found that 'habitual' cannabis users had a nine-fold higher crash risk that persisted after controlling for confounding factors including blood-alcohol concentration (BAC).

Studies of the effects of cannabis upon on-road driving performance have reported more modest impairments than comparable doses of alcohol

(Smiley, 1999). This appears to be because cannabis-intoxicated drivers drive more slowly and take fewer risks than alcohol-intoxicated drivers (Smiley, 1999). More recent studies on the effects of cannabis on driving performance on the road that have used doses closer to typical recreational doses (Robbe, 1994) have found small but consistent decrements in driving performance.

Cannabis is the illicit drug most often detected in the bodily fluids of drivers who have been injured or killed in motor vehicle crashes (see Kelly et al., 2004 for a review). It has been uncertain for a number of reasons whether cannabis has played a causal role in these accidents (Hall et al., 2001). First, earlier studies measured inactive cannabinoid metabolites in blood and urine, which only indicated that cannabis had been used within the past few days; they did not establish that the driver was intoxicated at the time of the accident (see Bates & Blakely, 1999; Hall et al., 2001; Kelly et al., 2004 for reviews). Secondly, many drivers with cannabinoids in their blood also had high blood alcohol levels (Bates & Blakely, 1999; Hall et al., 2001).

Better-controlled epidemiological studies have recently provided credible evidence that cannabis users who drive while intoxicated are at increased risk of motor vehicle crashes. Gerberich et al. (2003) found that current cannabis users had higher rates of hospitalization for injury from all causes than former cannabis users or non-users in a cohort of 64,657 patients from a Health Maintenance Organization. The relationship for motor vehicle accidents (relative risk (RR) = 1.96) persisted after statistical adjustment among men but not among women. Women in the cohort also had much lower rates of cannabis use and accidents. Mura et al. (2003) found a similar relationship in a study of THC in the serum of 900 persons hospitalized for motor vehicle injuries and 900 age-and-sex matched controls in France. They did not, however, statistically adjust for blood-alcohol level which was found in 40% of cases with THC present.

Drummer et al. (2004) assessed THC levels in blood in 1420 Australian drivers killed in accidents. They found that cannabis users were more likely to be culpable in accidents (odds ratio (OR) = 2.5) and there was a higher accident risk (OR = 6.6 [95% CI: 1.5, 28.0]) among those with THC levels greater than 5 ng/ml. Their findings differed from those of another Australian study (Longo et al., 2000) that did not find a relationship between THC and culpability. However, this study involved injuries rather than fatalities, there were longer delays between these accidents and drug testing, and the average levels of THC detected in blood were much lower than those reported by Drummer et al. (2004).

Laumon et al. (2005) compared blood THC levels in 6,766 culpable and 3,006 nonculpable drivers in France between October 2001 and September 2003.

There was an increased culpability for drivers with THC detected in their blood at levels of greater than 1 ng/ml (OR = 2.87). This increase was less than the 15.5 increase for drivers with BAC greater than 0.05 g/l. There was a dose-response relationship between THC and culpability that persisted after controlling for BAC, age, and time of accident. On these data, 2.5% of fatal accidents in France could be attributed to cannabis and 29% to alcohol (with a BAC of greater than 0.05%).

Bedard *et al.* (2007) examined the relationship between cannabis use and accident risk in 32,543 drivers killed in the United States between 1993 and 2003. They found a dose response relationship between BAC and culpability, and a more modest association (OR = 1.39 [99% CI: 1.21–1.59]) between culpability and cannabis use assessed in a variety of ways, including inactive metabolites. The association was attenuated but still significant after adjustment for crash history, age, convictions for drink driving and BAC (OR = 1.29).

A convergence of fallible evidence thus suggests that cannabis use increases the risk of motor vehicle crashes 2–3 times (Ramaekers *et al.*, 2004). The size of the effect on driving risks is much more modest than that of alcohol (with ORs for cannabis ranging from 1.3–3, compared with 6–15 for alcohol). The relationship may be attenuated because impairment is not as directly related to blood THC levels as is BAC. The estimated contribution of cannabis use to accident deaths has been much smaller than that of alcohol (2.5% vs. 29%). This probably reflects a combination of the lower crash risks in cannabis-impaired drivers and the lower prevalence of cannabis-impaired drivers.

The motor vehicle crash risks of cannabis use are of public health significance because of the high rates of cannabis use among young adults at highest risk of injury and death from car crashes. An additional concern is that the combined use of cannabis and alcohol (which is in some countries more common than cannabis use alone) probably increases the crash risk over that of either drug used on its own (Ramaekers *et al.*, 2004). The policy challenge is to define a level of THC in blood that can be used by courts to define impairment (Grotenhermen *et al.*, 2007).

Immunological effects

Cannabinoid CB_2 receptors are found in the immune system (Roth *et al.*, 2002), and animal studies suggest that high doses of cannabis extracts and of THC impair immune functioning. A number of studies in mice and guinea pigs suggest that high doses (200 mg/kg) of cannabinoids decrease resistance to infection with *Lysteria monocytogenes* (Morahan *et al.*, 1979) and *herpes simplex type 2* virus (e.g. Cabral & Pettit, 1998). There have, however, been very few epidemiological studies of immune system functioning and disease susceptibility in heavy cannabis users to assess how serious these immunological risks may be (Cabral & Pettit, 1998; Klein *et al.*, 2001; Roth *et al.*, 2002).

Several epidemiological studies have examined the effects of self-reported cannabis use on progression to AIDS among HIV-positive homosexual men. Kaslow *et al.* (1989) reported a prospective study of progression to AIDS among 4,954 HIV-positive homosexual and bisexual men. Cannabis use did not predict increased progression to AIDS, and it was not related to changes in immunological functioning. There was also no relationship between marijuana use and progression to AIDS in HIV-seropositive men in the San Francisco Men's Health Study (N = 451) over 6 years (DiFranco *et al.*, 1996). There was an increased risk of progression to AIDS among cannabis users in the Sydney AIDS Project, but the Institute of Medicine (Joy *et al.*, 1999) has described this finding as 'less reliable' than those of Kaslow *et al.* and DiFranco *et al.* because the study had a short follow-up period, and many of the 'HIV-positive cases' already had AIDS. A study of mortality among a cohort enrolled in a health insurance plan (Sidney *et al.*, 1997a) did find an association between cannabis use and death from AIDS, but this was attributed to confounding of cannabis use and sexual preference (which was not assessed in the study).

Reproductive effects of cannabis use

Cannabis is widely used by adolescents and young adults during the peak age for reproduction. Animal studies in the mid-1970s raised concerns that cannabis use during this period could adversely affect reproductive outcomes because large doses of THC reduced the secretion of gonadal hormones in both sexes (Brown & Dobs, 2002) and adversely affected foetal development (Bloch, 1983).

Effects on the male and female reproductive systems

In animals, marijuana, crude marijuana extracts, THC, and some purified cannabinoids depress male reproductive endocrine function (Bloch, 1983; Brown & Dobs, 2002). If used chronically, cannabis may reduce plasma testosterone, retard sperm maturation, reduce sperm count and sperm motility, and increase the rate of abnormal sperm production (Bloch, 1983; Murphy, 1999). The mechanisms for these effects are unclear but probably reflect the effects of THC on the testes, and indirectly on the hypothalamic hormones that stimulate the testes to produce testosterone (Brown & Dobs, 2002).

Studies of the effects of cannabis on human male reproductive function have produced mixed results (Brown & Dobs, 2002). An early study that reported reduced testosterone, sperm production, and sperm motility and increased abnormalities in sperm (Kolodny *et al.*, 1974) was not replicated in later studies (Brown & Dobs, 2002). The latter included a larger, well-controlled study on the effects of three weeks of daily cannabis use on plasma testosterone (Mendelson *et al.*, 1974). Other studies have produced both positive and negative evidence of an effect of cannabinoids on testosterone for reasons that are not well understood (Brown & Dobs, 2002). If there are effects of cannabis on male reproductive functioning, their clinical significance in humans is uncertain because testosterone levels have generally been within the normal range in studies that found effects (Hollister, 1986). A recent study of outcomes of in-vitro fertilization (IVF) and gamete intrafallopian transfer (GIFT) reported that males who reported using cannabis regularly fathered children with lower birth weights (Klonoff-Cohen *et al.*, 2006), although the mechanism for such an effect is unclear.

Animal studies also suggest that cannabis extracts and pure THC interfered with the hypothalamic-pituitary-gonadal axis in female rats (Bloch, 1983; Brown & Dobs, 2002), while chronic exposure delayed oestrous and ovulation (Murphy, 1999). There have been very few experimental studies on the effects of cannabis on the human female reproductive system, because of fears that cannabis use may produce birth defects in women of childbearing age. Mendelson and Mello (1984) observed hormonal levels in a group of female cannabis users (all of whom had undergone a tubal ligation) and failed to find any evidence that chronic cannabis use affected sex hormones or the duration of the cycle. A more recent observational study of the outcomes from in-vitro fertilization (IVF) and Gamete IntraFallopian Transfer (GIFT) found that women who had a history of past regular cannabis use had fewer oocytes retreived and fertilized than those who had not smoked cannabis (Klonoff-Cohen *et al.*, 2006).

Foetal development and birth defects

In animal studies very high doses of cannabis can produce resorption, growth retardation, and malformations in mice, rats, rabbits, and hamsters (Bloch, 1983). Birth malformations have been observed more often after crude marijuana extract rather than THC, suggesting that other cannabinoids may have teratogenic effects. Bloch (1983) concluded that THC was unlikely to be teratogenic in humans because 'the few reports of teratogenicity in rodents and rabbits indicate that cannabinoids are, at most, weakly teratogenic in these species' (p. 416).

Epidemiological studies on the effects of cannabis use on human development have produced mixed results for a number of reasons. First, heavy cannabis use is relatively rare during pregnancy, so very large sample sizes are needed to detect any adverse effects on foetal development (Fried & Smith, 2001).

Many of the studies have been too small to detect such effects. Secondly, the stigma of admitting to drugs use during pregnancy encourages under-reporting (Day *et al.*, 1985). If a substantial proportion of cannabis users are misclassified as non-users, any relationship between cannabis use and adverse outcomes will be attenuated. Thirdly, there are difficulties in interpreting associations that have been reported between adverse pregnancy outcomes and cannabis use (e.g. Forrester & Merz, 2007) because cannabis users are also more likely to use tobacco, alcohol, and other illicit drugs during pregnancy (Eyler & Behnke, 1999), and they are also less likely to seek antenatal care and more likely to have poorer nutrition than women who do not use cannabis (Tennes *et al.*, 1985).

Cannabis use in pregnancy is more consistently associated with reduced birth weight (Fergusson *et al.*, 2002a; Gibson *et al.*, 1983; Hatch & Bracken, 1986; Zuckerman *et al.*, 1989). This relationship was found in one of the largest, best-controlled studies (e.g. Fergusson *et al.*, 2002a), where it persisted after statistically controlling for confounding variables (e.g. Fergusson et al., 2002a; Hatch & Bracken, 1986; Zuckerman *et al.*, 1989). A meta-analysis of these studies (English *et al.*, 1997) found that regular cannabis-smoking during pregnancy reduced birth weight, though less than tobacco-smoking.

There has been no consistent relationship between cannabis use and birth abnormalities. Early case reports of birth abnormalities in children born to women who had smoked cannabis during pregnancy have generally not been supported by epidemiological studies (Gibson *et al.*, 1983; Hingson *et al.*, 1982a; Tennes *et al.*, 1985; Zuckerman *et al.*, 1989). One recent study found associations between cannabis use during pregnancy and a large number of birth defects in infants born in Hawaii between 1986 and 2002 (Forrester & Merz, 2007), but the study was unable to control for important confounding variables. Zuckerman *et al.* (1989) failed to find an increased risk of birth defects. This was a convincing negative finding because they studied a large sample of women among whom there was a substantial rate of cannabis use that was verified by urinalysis. There was a low rate of birth abnormalities among the cannabis users, and no suggestion of an increase by comparison with the controls.

Post-natal effects of intrauterine exposure to cannabinoids

The Ontario Prospective Prenatal Study (OPPS) has studied developmental and behavioural abnormalities in children born to women who reported using cannabis during pregnancy (Fried & Smith, 2001; Fried & Watkinson, 2000; Hutchings & Fried, 1999). In this study, mothers were asked about their drug use during pregnancy and their children were measured on the Brazelton scales after birth, neurologically assessed at one month, and again at six and twelve months.

There was some developmental delay shortly after birth in the visual system, and increased tremor and startle among the children of cannabis users (Fried & Smith, 2001), but these behavioural effects faded by one month, and no differences were detected on ability tests at six and twelve months. Subtle behavioural effects of cannabis were subsequently reported at 36 and 48 months, but not at 60 and 72 months (Fried & Smith, 2001). These results are suggestive of a subtle developmental impairment occurring among children who had experienced a shorter gestation and prematurity (Fried & Smith, 2001). The cohort has now been followed up to age 9–12 years. No differences were found between children who were and were not exposed to cannabis during pregnancy on full-scale IQ scores, but there were small differences in measures of perceptual organization and higher cognitive processes (Fried & Smith, 2001).

Attempts to replicate these OPPS findings have been mixed. Tennes *et al.* (1985) studied the relationship between cannabis use during pregnancy and postnatal development of the child in 756 women, a third of whom reported cannabis use during pregnancy. They found no evidence of impaired development of the visual system, no increased risk of tremor or startle at birth, and no differences at 1 year between the children of users and nonusers. Day *et al.* (1994), by contrast, followed up children at age three who were born to 655 teenage women in Pittsburgh between 1990 and 1995. They found poorer performances on memory and verbal scales of the Stanford-Binet Intelligence Scale at age three in children of women who reported cannabis use during pregnancy. At age six, prenatal cannabis exposure was associated with reduced height, after controlling for alcohol and tobacco use and other predictors of impaired growth (Cornelius *et al.*, 2002). By age 10, antenatal cannabis exposure was associated with increased delinquency and problem behaviour (Goldschmidt *et al.*, 2000).

Overall, the post-natal behavioural effects of prenatal cannabis exposure appear to be modest (Huizink & Mulder, 2006). Their existence remains uncertain because of the small size of the effects and their tendency to come and go at different ages. The causal interpretation of the effects reported is complicated by the inability of these studies to adequately control for confounding variables (Huizink & Mulder, 2006), such as other drug use during pregnancy, poor parenting skills, and shared genetic risks for impaired cognitive functioning in both mothers and their infants.

Maternal cannabis use and childhood cancers

Cannabis smoking has also been linked with cancers among children born to mothers who used cannabis during pregnancy in three case-control studies.

In none was there an *a priori* reason to expect a relationship between cannabis use and these cancers.

An association between maternal cannabis use and childhood cancer was reported in a case-control study of Acute Nonlymphoblastic Leukemia (ANLL) (Neglia *et al.*, 1991; Robinson *et al.*, 1989). Maternal cannabis use was assessed as a potential confounder. Mothers of cases were 11 times more likely to have used cannabis before and during their pregnancy than were the mothers of controls. The relationship persisted after statistical adjustment for other risk factors. Reporting bias was an alternative explanation because the reports of cannabis use were obtained after diagnosis of ANLL and the rate of cannabis use was lower in controls than in general population surveys. Two other case-control studies have reported an increased risk of rhabdomyosarcoma (Grufferman *et al.*, 1993) and astrocytomas (Kuijten *et al.*, 1992) in children born to women who reported using cannabis during their pregnancies. In each study, cannabis use was one of a large number of confounding variables that were measured. The possibility of measurement bias in these studies was quite high (Hashibe *et al.*, 2005).

There have been no increases in the incidence of these childhood cancers over the period 1979–1995 that could be explained by increased maternal cannabis use during pregnancy (Reis *et al.*, 2000). The incidence of ANLL, for example, remained steady between 1979 and 1995 (Smith *et al.*, 2000) despite the very high relative risk reported for this cancer. The same was true for soft-tissue sarcomas (which include rhabdomyosarcomas) (Gurney *et al.*, 2000b). Central nervous system (CNS) malignancies (about 52% of which are astrocytomas) increased in incidence between 1979 and 1995 (Gurney *et al.*, 2000a) but in a way that was unlikely to reflect maternal cannabis use. Incidence was steady between 1979 and 1985, when it abruptly increased, and it remained steady thereafter (Gurney *et al.*, 2000a). Magnetic resonance imaging (MRI) became widely used in the United States in 1985, which suggests that the increase was an artefact of improved diagnosis rather than an increase in incidence (Gurney *et al.*, 2000a).

The health effects of chronic cannabis use

'Chronic' cannabis use is a broad term meant to cover the regular (especially daily or near daily) use over periods of years. Epidemiological studies of relationships between chronic cannabis use and various human diseases are now being conducted. There are problems with these studies in assessing exposure to cannabis over extended periods and excluding alternative explanations of the associations. A major problem in interpreting epidemiological studies is that cannabis use is correlated with other drug use which is known to adversely affect health (e.g. alcohol and tobacco use). Generally, the heavier the cannabis use, the more likely it is that the person uses other licit (alcohol and tobacco) and illicit drugs (amphetamines, hallucinogens, cocaine, and heroin). This makes it difficult to confidently attribute some of the adverse health effects found in cannabis users to their cannabis use (Hall, 1999). Statistical control of confounding variables is the best available approach to deal with this problem.

In the following sections we discuss the evidence on the adverse health and psychological effects that have been most commonly attributed to regular cannabis use. We begin with the question of whether cannabis is a drug of dependence, and then consider the most plausible adverse physical health effects of chronic use, namely respiratory and cardiovascular disease. We end by exploring the evidence on the adverse psychological effects that chronic cannabis use may have on adolescent development and the mental health of young adults via psychosis, depressive disorders, and cognitive impairment.

Cannabis dependence

Both the Diagnostic and Statistical Manual of Mental Disorders (DSM-IV-TR) and the International Classification of Diseases (ICD-10) include a diagnosis of cannabis dependence that is characterized by marked distress resulting from a recurring cluster of problems that reflect impaired control over cannabis use and continued cannabis use despite harms arising from its use. Community mental health surveys indicate that in many developed societies cannabis dependence is the most common type of drug dependence after alcohol and tobacco (Anthony & Helzer, 1991; Hall et al., 1999b; Kessler et al., 1994; Stinson et al., 2006). About 2% of adults meet criteria for cannabis abuse and dependence in the past year (Stinson et al., 2006; Swift et al., 2001), with a lifetime rate of 4–8% in US adults (Anthony & Helzer, 1991; Stinson et al., 2006). The risk of dependence is around 9% among persons who have ever used cannabis (Anthony et al., 1994; Swift et al., 2001) and around one in six for young people who initiate in adolescence (Swift et al., 2001). These risks compare with risks of 32% for nicotine, 23% for heroin, 17% for cocaine, 15% for alcohol, and 11% for stimulant users (Anthony et al., 1994). Those at highest risk of cannabis dependence have a history of poor academic achievement, deviant behaviour in childhood and adolescence, nonconformity and rebelliousness, poor parental relationships, and a parental history of drug and alcohol problems (Coffey et al., 2003; Swift et al., 2001).

Animals and humans develop tolerance to many of the behavioural and physiological effects of THC (Lichtman & Martin, 2005; Maldonado, 2002).

The cannabinoid antagonist SR 141716A precipitates a withdrawal syndrome in rats, mice, and dogs (e.g. Selley *et al.*, 2003) that is reversed by administering THC (Lichtman *et al.*, 2001). Down-regulation of CB1 receptors may underlie the development of tolerance (Lichtman & Martin, 2005).

Similar withdrawal symptoms occur in humans (Budney & Hughes, 2006). This includes subjects abruptly withdrawn after 30 days on high dose THC (Jones *et al.*, 1976), and chronic recreational cannabis users (Kouri & Pope, 2000), including such users who were not seeking help to stop use (Budney *et al.*, 2001). Long-term users seeking help to stop often report withdrawal symptoms that include anxiety, insomnia, appetite disturbance, and depression (Budney & Hughes, 2006; Budney *et al.*, 2004), and they also report using cannabis to relieve withdrawal symptoms (Budney *et al.*, 2007).

Over the past two decades, increasing numbers of cannabis users have sought help in the United States, Europe, and Australia because of difficulties they experienced in stopping their cannabis use (AIHW, 2006; EMCDDA, 2003; SAMHSA, 2004). Some have argued that this increase is the result of increased diversion of cannabis users into treatment by the courts (Zimmer & Morgan, 1997). This seems less likely to explain similar increases in the Netherlands, where the use of cannabis is de-facto largely decriminalized (Dutch National Alcohol and Drug Information System, 2006).

Cannabis dependence can be treated on an outpatient basis using cognitive-behavioural therapy (CBT) (McRae *et al.*, 2003). CBT reduces cannabis use and cannabis-related problems (Denis *et al.*, 2006; McRae *et al.*, 2003), although the proportion of those who achieve enduring abstinence is modest (Denis *et al.*, 2006). Continuous abstinence rates have been as low as 15% 6–12 months after treatment (Copeland *et al.*, 2001; Denis *et al.*, 2006), with the best abstinence rate (35%) reported from combined CBT and contingency management using vouchers in a sample of 20 patients (McRae *et al.*, 2003). Pharmacological efforts to improve the management of cannabis withdrawal symptoms (Kleber *et al.*, 2007) have not to date found any agent superior to placebo (Budney & Hughes, 2006; Hart, 2005).

The respiratory risks of cannabis smoking

Over the past two decades, cross-sectional and longitudinal studies in the United States (Tashkin *et al.*, 2002) and New Zealand (Aldington *et al.*, 2007; Taylor *et al.*, 2000; 2002), have shown that people who are regular smokers of cannabis have more symptoms of chronic bronchitis (wheeze, sputum production, and chronic coughs) than non-smokers (see Tashkin *et al.*, 2002; Tetrault *et al.*, 2007 for reviews). The immunological competence of the respiratory system in people who only smoke cannabis is also impaired, increasing their susceptibility to respiratory infections and pneumonia, and their use of health services for these infections (Tashkin et al., 2002).

The effects of long-term cannabis smoking on respiratory function are less clear (Tashkin et al., 2002; Tetrault et al., 2007). A longitudinal study (Taylor et al., 2000; 2002) of respiratory function in 1,037 New Zealand youths followed from birth until the age of 21 (Taylor et al., 2000) and 26 (Taylor et al., 2002) found that cannabis-dependent subjects had impaired respiratory function. But this finding has not been replicated in a longer follow-up study of Tashkin's cohort (Tashkin et al., 2002).

There is no evidence to date that chronic cannabis smoking increases the risk of emphysema (Tashkin, 2005). Follow-up studies of Tashkin's cohort after 8 years failed to find increased rates of emphysema in marijuana-only smokers (Tashkin, 2005). The same result has recently been reported in a similarly recruited group of heavy cannabis-only smokers in New Zealand (Aldington et al., 2007).

Respiratory cancers

There are good reasons for believing that cannabis can cause cancers of the lung and the aerodigestive tract (Hall & MacPhee, 2002; Hashibe et al., 2005). Cannabis smoke contains many of the same carcinogens as tobacco smoke, which is a cause of respiratory cancer (Hashibe et al., 2005; Marselos & Karamanakos, 1999). Some of these carcinogens occur at higher levels in cannabis than tobacco smoke (Moir et al., 2008). Cannabis smoke is mutagenic in the Ames test and causes cancers in the mouse skin test (MacPhee, 1999; Marselos & Karamanakos, 1999). Cannabis smokers inhale more deeply than tobacco smokers, retaining more tar and particulate matter (Hashibe et al., 2005; Tashkin, 1999); and chronic cannabis smokers show many of the pathological changes in lung cells that precede the development of cancer in tobacco smokers (Tashkin, 1999).

The results of epidemiological studies of upper respiratory tract cancers in cannabis users have been mixed. Sidney et al. (1997b) studied cancer incidence in an 8.6-year follow-up of 64,855 members of the Kaiser Permanente Medical Care Program. There was no increased risk of respiratory cancer at follow-up among those who had ever used cannabis and current cannabis users. Males who had smoked cannabis had an increased risk of prostate cancer (RR = 3.1), and so did current cannabis smokers (RR = 4.7).

Zhang et al. (1999), by contrast, found an increased risk of squamous cell carcinoma of the head and neck among cannabis users in a case-control study of 173 persons with this cancer and 176 controls (blood donors matched on age and sex from the same hospital). There was an odds ratio of 2 for cannabis smoking after adjusting for cigarette smoking, alcohol use, and other risk factors. Two other case-control studies of oral squamous cell carcinoma, however, have failed to find any association between cannabis use and oral cancers. Llewellyn *et al.* (2004) failed to find any association between self-reported cannabis use and oral cancers in a study of 116 cases (identified from a cancer register) and 207 age- and sex-matched controls (sampled from the same general practices as the cases). Rosenblatt *et al.* also reported a null finding in a community-based study of 407 cases and 615 controls aged 18 to 65 years in Washington State (Rosenblatt *et al.*, 2004).

Case-control studies of cannabis smoking and lung cancer have produced more consistent evidence of harm (Mehra *et al.*, 2006). A Tunisian case-control study of 110 cases of hospital-diagnosed lung cancer and 110 community controls found an association with cannabis use (OR = 8.2) that persisted after adjustment for cigarette smoking, water pipe, and snuff use. A Moroccan case-control study of 118 cases and 235 control subjects also found an increased risk of lung cancer (OR = 5.6) among those who smoked a combination of cannabis flowers and tobacco but a more marginal relationship for those who only smoked cannabis. A New Zealand case-control study of lung cancer in 79 adults under the age of 55 years and 324 community controls (Aldington *et al.*, 2008) reported a dose-response relationship between lung cancer risks and frequency of cannabis use. Among the highest third of cannabis users there was a 5.7 times higher risk of lung cancer.

Uncertainties remain about the risk of oral and respiratory cancers among cannabis smokers (Hashibe *et al.*, 2005; Mehra *et al.*, 2006). The risk of oral cancer is small compared to that for tobacco smoking, given the small relative risk in the only positive study (Rosenblatt *et al.*, 2004). The findings from the case-control studies of lung cancer are more suggestive of higher risks, but the measures of cannabis use in these studies have been relatively crude and it is unclear how well these studies have been able to control for tobacco smoking. Larger cohort studies and better-designed case-control studies of tobacco-related cancers are needed to clarify the relationship between cannabis smoking and the risks of these cancers (Hall & MacPhee, 2002; Mehra *et al.*, 2006).

Cardiovascular effects of cannabis smoking

In humans and animals, cannabis and THC produce dose-related increases in heart rate (Chesher & Hall, 1999; Jones, 2002). The hearts of healthy young adults are only mildly stressed by this effect and tolerance develops quickly (Joy *et al.*, 1999; Jones, 2002; Sidney, 2002). There are more reasons for concern about these effects in older adults, who are at increased risk of ischaemic heart disease, hypertension, and cerebrovascular disease (Jones, 2002; Sidney, 2002).

There are case reports of myocardial infarction, arrythmias, and vascular complications in young otherwise healthy cannabis users (Aryana & Williams, 2007), but there have been few epidemiological or other controlled studies.

A case-crossover study by Mittleman *et al.* (2001) of 3,882 patients who had had a myocardial infarction suggested that cannabis use increased the risk of a myocardial infarction 4.8 times in the hour after use (compared with 24-fold for cocaine). Mittleman *et al.* estimated that a 44-year-old adult who used cannabis daily would increase his or her annual risk of an acute cardiovascular event by 1.5–3%. Mukamal *et al.* (2008) recently provided support for Mittleman *et al.* in a prospective study of 1,913 adults hospitalized for myocardial infarction. They found a dose-response relationship between self-reported cannabis use at baseline and mortality over the subsequent 3.8 years. The mortality risk increased 2.5 times for less-than-weekly users, and 4.2 times for more-than-weekly users. Both sets of findings are supported by double-blind laboratory studies which show that smoking cannabis produces symptoms of angina in patients with heart disease (Aronow & Cassidy, 1974; 1975; Gottschalk *et al.*, 1977).

Chronic cannabis use and brain function

Cognitive functioning

Cognitive impairment, particularly in short-term memory, is often reported by cannabis-dependent persons seeking help to stop using cannabis (Solowij, 1998). Controlled studies have not found that long-term use produces *severe* impairment of cognitive function (Solowij, 1998). Lyketsos *et al.* (1999) assessed cognitive decline on the Mini Mental State Examination (MMSE) in 1,318 adults over 11.5 years. They found no relationship between cannabis use and decline in MMSE score, indicating that cannabis use did not produce *gross* cognitive impairment (Solowij, 1998). This study does not exclude the possibility of more subtle cognitive impairment, because the MMSE is a screening test that is not sensitive to small changes in cognitive functions, and in this study 'heavy cannabis users' included anyone who ever reported smoking daily for more than 2 weeks.

There is evidence from controlled laboratory studies that long-term heavy cannabis users show more subtle types of cognitive impairment (Solowij, 1998). A major problem in interpreting these studies has been excluding the possibility that regular cannabis users had poorer cognitive functioning than controls before they started to use cannabis (Solowij, 1998). The better studies have matched users and non-users on estimated premorbid intellectual functioning (Solowij, 1998) or on cognitive test performance before the onset of cannabis use (e.g. Block *et al.*, 2002). These have found cognitive impairments associated with frequent and/or long term cannabis use (Block & Ghoneim, 1993; Block *et al.*, 2002).

Solowij *et al.* (2002), for example, found little impairment in the neuro-psychological performance of dependent, heavy cannabis users (near daily) with an average 10 years of regular use when compared to nonuser controls. Users with an average of 24 years of regular use, however, showed impaired attention and impaired verbal learning, retention, and retrieval. Solowij (1998) used event-related potentials to show impaired attention in shorter term users (5+ years) and found that impairment increased with the number of years of cannabis use (Solowij, 1998; 2002).

Deficits in verbal learning, memory, and attention are the most consistently replicated impairments in heavy cannabis users. There is disagreement about their explanation. They have been variously related to duration (Solowij *et al.*, 2002), frequency (Pope *et al.*, 2001), and cumulative dosage of THC (Bolla *et al.*, 2002). The differential effects of frequency and duration of use and dose reported in some studies have not always been reported. Debate continues on the issue of whether these deficits are attributable to lingering acute drug effects, drug residues, abstinence effects, or gradual changes in the brain as a result of cumulative THC exposure (Pope *et al.*, 1995; Solowij *et al.*, 2002).

It is also uncertain whether cognitive functioning recovers after cessation of cannabis use. Solowij (1998) found partial recovery on a selective attention task after 2 years' abstinence in a small group of ex-users, but brain event-related potential measures continued to show impaired information-processing, the severity of which was correlated with the years of cannabis use. Bolla *et al.* (2002) found persistent dose-related decrements in neurocognitive perform-ance after 28 days of abstinence in heavy young users (mean age of 20 and 5 years use), while Pope *et al.* (2001) reported that memory impairments recovered after 28 days of abstinence. Another report on the latter sample (Pope *et al.*, 2002) found persistent memory deficits in those who had started using before the age of 17.

Brain structure and function

An early finding of structural brain changes after prolonged cannabis use was not replicated (see Solowij, 1998; 1999 for reviews). One study used sophisti-cated measurement techniques to show that frequent but relatively short-term use of cannabis produced neither structural brain abnormalities nor global or regional changes in brain tissue volume or composition that are assessed by MRI (Block *et al.*, 2000a). Other research has found reduced cortical grey matter and increased white matter in those who commenced using cannabis before age 17 compared to those who started using later (Wilson *et al.*, 2000). It remains uncertain whether these findings reflect a cause or a consequence of early cannabis use.

A number of more recent studies have demonstrated altered brain function and metabolism in humans following acute and chronic use of cannabis using cerebral blood flow (CBF), PET, and electroencephalographic (EEG) techniques. Block and colleagues (2000b), for example, found that after 26 hours of supervised abstinence, regular cannabis users showed substantially lower resting brain–blood flow than controls in the posterior cerebellum and prefrontal cortex. Similarly, Lundqvist *et al.* (2001) showed lower mean hemispheric and frontal blood flow shortly after cessation of cannabis use. It remains to be determined whether these findings have any longer term implications for cognitive functioning.

Loeber and Yurgelun-Todd (1999) have proposed that chronic cannabis use changes the cannabinoid receptors that act on the dopamine system, producing a reduction in brain metabolism in the frontal lobe and cerebellum. Recent studies using functional imaging techniques during cognitive tasks (e.g. Porrino *et al.*, 2004; Quickfall & Crockford, 2006; Smith *et al.*, 2004; Solowij *et al.*, 2004) have shown diminished activity in the brains of chronic cannabis users compared to controls, even after cannabis users had abstained for 28 days (Block *et al.*, 2002; Loeber & Yurgelun-Todd, 1999).

Changes in cannabinoid receptor activity in the hippocampus, prefrontal cortex and cerebellum have also been implicated in the cognitive impairments associated with chronic cannabis use. Yücel *et al.* (2008) recently reported reductions in the volumes of the hippocampus and amygdala in 15 long-term users who had smoked 5 or more joints a day for 10 or more years. The size of the reductions was also correlated with the duration of use. More functional brain imaging studies of this type on larger samples of long-term users hold the most promise in investigating whether the cognitive impairment found in long-term users is correlated with structural changes in areas of the brain that are implicated in memory and emotion and also richly endowed with cannabinoid receptors (Solowij *et al.*, 2004).

The consequences of adolescent cannabis use

Cannabis first began to be used by large numbers of young people in the United States in the early 1970s. In the decades since then, the proportion of young people who have used cannabis in many developed countries has increased, and age of first use has fallen in Australia, the United States, and the Netherlands (Hall & Pacula, 2003). There has been considerable community concern about whether adolescent cannabis use increases poor educational outcomes (Lynskey & Hall, 2000), the use of heroin and cocaine (Fergusson *et al.*, 2002b), and psychosis (Hall & Pacula, 2003).

Educational outcomes

Cannabis use acutely impairs memory and attention. Its regular use could potentially adversely affect learning in adolescents, producing poorer school performance and increasing early school drop out. Surveys typically find associations between cannabis use and poor educational attainment among school children and youth (e.g. Lifrak *et al.*, 1997; Resnick *et al.*, 1997; see Lynskey & Hall, 2000 for a review). Rates of cannabis use are also higher among young people who no longer attend school or who had high rates of absenteeism when at school (Fergusson *et al.*, 1996; Lynskey *et al.*, 1999).

One explanation of these associations is that cannabis use is a contributory cause of poor school performance (e.g. Kandel *et al.*, 1986). A second possibility is that heavy cannabis use is a consequence of poor educational attainment (Hawkins *et al.*, 1992). The first and second hypotheses could both be true if, for example, poor school performance increased cannabis use which in turn further impaired school performance. A third hypothesis is that cannabis use and poor educational attainment are the result of common factors that increase the risk of both early cannabis use and poor educational performance (Donovan & Jessor, 1985). This hypothesis is supported by the overlap between risk factors for early cannabis use and poor educational performance (see Hawkins *et al.*, 1992 for reviews).

These explanations can only be distinguished by prospective studies of young people who are assessed over time on their cannabis use, educational attainment and potentially confounding factors, such as family and social circumstances, personality characteristics, and delinquency (Lynskey & Hall, 2000). Such studies enable researchers to answer the question: do young people who use cannabis have poorer educational outcomes than those who do not, when we allow for the fact that cannabis users are more likely to have a history of poor school performance and other characteristics before they used cannabis?

Longitudinal studies (e.g. Fergusson *et al.*, 1996) have typically found a relationship between cannabis use before the age of 15 years and early school leaving. This has persisted after statistical adjustment for differences between early cannabis users and their peers (e.g. Duncan *et al.*, 1998; Ellickson *et al.*, 1998; Tanner *et al.*, 1999). The most plausible hypothesis seems to be that the impaired educational performance in adolescent cannabis users is attributable to a higher pre-existing risk of these outcomes and a combination of the effects of acute intoxication upon cognitive performance, affiliation with peers who reject school, and a desire to make an early transition to adulthood (Lynskey & Hall, 2000). This hypothesis is supported by the lack of any relationship between marijuana use and dropping out of university in a longitudinal study of male American university students; among men who had used marijuana but no other drugs, 'there was no evidence that drug use had any relation to dropping out that was independent of family background, relationships with parents in high school, and social values' (Mellinger *et al.*, 1976).

Other illicit drug use

Surveys of adolescent drug use in the United States over the past 30 years have consistently shown three relationships between cannabis and the use of heroin and cocaine (see Kandel, 2002 for a review). First, almost all of those who tried cocaine and heroin first used alcohol, tobacco, and cannabis. Second, regular cannabis users were more likely to later use heroin and cocaine. Third, the earlier the age at which cannabis was first used, the more likely a user was to use heroin and cocaine. These relationships have been confirmed in longitudinal studies of drug use in New Zealand (Fergusson & Horwood, 2000; McGee & Feehan, 1993).

Three types of explanation have been offered for these patterns of drug involvement. The first is that because cannabis and other illicit drugs are supplied by the same black market, cannabis users have more opportunities to use other illicit drugs than non-cannabis users (Cohen, 1976). The second hypothesis is that those who are early cannabis users are more likely to use other illicit drugs for reasons unrelated to their cannabis use (Morral *et al.*, 2002). The third hypothesis is that the pharmacological effects of cannabis increase the propensity to use other illicit drugs (Murray *et al.*, 2007).

Social environment and drug availability do play a role. Young people in the United States who have used alcohol or tobacco are more likely to report opportunities to use cannabis at an earlier age than those who have not (Wagner & Anthony, 2002). Moreover, those who had used cannabis reported more opportunities to use cocaine at an earlier age (Wagner & Anthony, 2002). In New Zealand, however, self-reported affiliation with drug-using peers only partially explained the relationship between cannabis and other illicit drug use (Fergusson & Horwood, 2000).

There is also evidence that socially deviant young people who have a predilection to use a variety of drugs including alcohol, cannabis, cocaine, and heroin are selectively recruited to cannabis use (Fergusson & Horwood, 2000). The sequence of drug involvement, on this hypothesis, reflects the differing availability and societal disapproval of cannabis and other illicit drug use (Donovan & Jessor, 1983). The selective recruitment hypothesis is supported by correlations between dropping out of high school, early premarital sexual experience, delinquency, and early alcohol- and illicit drug-use. Regular cannabis users are more likely than their peers to have a history of all these behaviours (Hawkins *et al.*, 1992; McGee & Feehan, 1993). The selective recruitment hypothesis has also been supported by a simulation study by Morral *et al.* (2002) which showed that this model could reproduce all the relationships between cannabis and other illicit drug use described above.

The selective recruitment hypothesis has been tested in longitudinal studies by assessing whether cannabis users are more likely to report heroin and cocaine use after statistically controlling for differences between them and nonusers (e.g. Fergusson *et al.*, 2002b; Kandel *et al.*, 1986; Lessem *et al.*, 2006; Yamaguchi & Kandel, 1984). Generally, adjustment for these pre-existing differences weakens but has not eliminated the strong relationships between early and regular cannabis use and an increased risk of using other illicit drugs (see Hall & Lynskey, 2005 for a review).

Behaviour genetic studies have tested an alternative explanation of the association between cannabis and other illicit drug use: that there is a shared genetic vulnerability to develop dependence on cannabis and other drugs (Agrawal *et al.*, 2007). Studies of identical and non-identical twins indicate that there is a partially shared genetic vulnerability to dependence on alcohol (Heath, 1995), cannabis (Agrawal & Lynskey, 2006), and tobacco (Han *et al.*, 1999; True *et al.*, 1999). Lynskey *et al.* (2003) tested this hypothesis by assessing the relationship between cannabis and other illicit drug use in 136 monozygotic and 175 dizygotic twin pairs in which one twin had, and the other twin had not, used cannabis before the age of 17 years. They found that the twin who had used cannabis was more likely to have used sedatives, hallucinogens, stimulants, and opioids than their co-twin who had not. These relationships persisted after controlling for environmental factors that predicted an increased risk of developing drug abuse or dependence. A similar finding has been reported in a study of Dutch twins (Lynskey *et al.*, 2006).

Animal studies suggest a number of ways in which the pharmacological effects of cannabis use could predispose cannabis users to use other illicit drugs (Nahas, 1990). First, cannabis, cocaine, heroin, and nicotine all act on the same brain 'reward centre' in the nucleus accumbens (Gardner, 1999). Secondly, the cannabinoid and opioid systems in the brain interact with each other (Manzanares *et al.*, 1999; Tanda *et al.*, 1997). Thirdly, mutant mice in which the cannabinoid receptor had been 'knocked out' do not find opioids rewarding (Ledent *et al.*, 1999).

Animal studies also potentially provide direct tests on whether these neural mechanisms may explain the relationship between cannabis and other illicit drug use in humans. Specifically, they can assess whether administration of cannabinoids 'primes' animals to self-administer other illicit drugs (Zimmer & Morgan, 1997). Two studies in rats (Cadoni *et al.*, 2001; Lamarque *et al.*, 2001), for example, have provided some evidence for cross-sensitivity between cannabinoids and opioids (Lamarque *et al.*, 2001). Their relevance to adolescent cannabis use is uncertain, however, because these effects were produced by injecting large doses of cannabinoids (Lynskey, 2002).

Cannabis use is more strongly associated with other illicit drug use than alcohol or tobacco use, and the earliest and most frequent cannabis users are the most likely to use other illicit drugs. Animal studies provide some biological plausibility for a causal relationship between cannabis and other types of illicit drug use. Well-controlled longitudinal studies suggest that selective recruitment to cannabis use does not wholly explain the association between cannabis use and the use of other illicit drugs. This is supported by discordant twin studies which suggest that shared genes and environment do not wholly explain the association. Nonetheless, it has been difficult to exclude the hypothesis that the pattern of use reflects the common characteristics of those who use cannabis and other drugs (Macleod *et al.*, 2004).

Cannabis use and mental health

Psychosis and schizophrenia

Cannabis use and psychotic symptoms are associated in general population surveys (see Degenhardt & Hall, 2006 for a review), and the relationship persists after adjusting for confounders (e.g. Degenhardt & Hall, 2001). The best evidence that these associations may be causal comes from longitudinal studies of large representative cohorts.

One of the earliest prospective studies of cannabis use and schizophrenia was a 15-year follow-up of 50,465 Swedish conscripts. It found that those who had tried cannabis by age 18 were 2.4 times more likely to be diagnosed with schizophrenia than those who had not (Andréasson *et al.*, 1987). The risk increased with the frequency of cannabis use. Although substantially reduced, it remained significant after statistical adjustment for confounding variables. Those who had used cannabis 10 or more times by age 18 were 2.3 times more likely to receive a diagnosis of schizophrenia than those who had not.

Zammit *et al.* (2002) reported a 27-year follow-up study of the same Swedish cohort. They found a dose-response relationship between frequency of cannabis use at age 18 and risk of schizophrenia during the follow-up. They also demonstrated that the relationship persisted after statistically controlling for the effects of other drug use and other potential confounding factors.

They estimated that 13% of cases of schizophrenia could be averted if all cannabis use were prevented.

Zammit *et al.*'s findings have been supported by other longitudinal studies. A three-year longitudinal study of the relationship between self-reported cannabis use and psychosis in a sample of 4,848 people in the Netherlands (van Os *et al.*, 2002) found a dose-response relationship between cannabis use at baseline and psychotic symptoms during the follow-up period that persisted after statistically controlling for the effects of other drug use. Henquet *et al.* (2004) reported a 4-year follow-up of a cohort of 2,437 adolescents and young adults between 1995 and 1999 in Munich, which found a dose-response relationship between self-reported cannabis use at baseline and the likelihood of reporting psychotic symptoms at follow up. Arseneault *et al.* (2002) found a relationship between cannabis use by age 15 and an increased risk of psychotic symptoms by age 26 in a prospective study of a New Zealand birth cohort. Fergusson *et al.* (2003) reported similar findings in a longitudinal study of the Christchurch birth cohort in New Zealand. Cannabis dependence at age 18 predicted an increased risk of psychotic symptoms at age 21 years (RR of 2.3), which was reduced but still significant after adjustment for potential confounders (RR of 1.8).

Moore *et al.* (2007) conducted a meta-analysis of these longitudinal studies and reported an odds ratio of 1.4 [95% CI: 1.20, 1.65] of psychotic disorder among those who had ever used cannabis. There was also a dose-response relationship between frequency of cannabis use and the risk of developing psychotic symptoms or a psychotic disorder. Reverse causation was controlled in the majority of these studies by either excluding cases reporting psychotic symptoms at baseline or by statistically adjusting for pre-existing psychotic symptoms. The common causal hypothesis was harder to exclude in all studies; the association between cannabis use and psychosis was attenuated after statistical adjustment for some potential confounders, and no study assessed all major potential confounders.

Has the incidence of schizophrenia, particularly early-onset acute cases, changed over the period when there have been very substantial increases in cannabis use among young adults in Australia and North America? A study modelling trends in the incidence of psychoses in Australia did not find clear evidence of an increase in incidence following steep increases in cannabis use during the 1980s (Degenhardt *et al.*, 2003). A similar study in Britain (Hickman *et al.*, 2007) suggested that it may be too early to detect any effect that cannabis use has on the incidence of psychoses in the United Kingdom, because its use only increased during the 1990s. The latter study estimated that in order to prevent one case of schizophrenia in British men aged 20–24, we would need to prevent 5,000 men from ever smoking cannabis. The evidence from recent studies attempting to detect an increase has been mixed: one British (Boydell *et al.*, 2006) and a Swiss study (Ajdacic-Gross *et al.*, 2007) reported increased incidence of psychoses among males in recent birth cohorts but another British study did not find any increase (Advisory Council on the Misuse of Drugs, 2008).

A study that found an interaction between cannabis use and a common polymorphism in the COMT Val[158]Met allele has suggested a biological basis for the relationship between cannabis use and psychosis (Caspi *et al.*, 2005). Alterations in catecholamine, particularly dopamine, metabolism have been documented in persons with schizophrenia (Bilder *et al.*, 2004), and the COMT functional polymorphism is very important for the metabolism of dopamine (Mannisto & Kaakkola, 2006). This suggestive finding has not been replicated, however, in a larger case-control study of schizophrenia and cannabis use in the United Kingdom (Zammit *et al.*, 2007).

There is also some experimental support for a direct effect of cannabis on psychotic symptoms from a provocation study by D'Souza *et al.* (D'Souza, 2004; 2005; 2007). In this study intravenous THC given under double-blind placebo controlled conditions produced dose-dependent increases in positive and negative psychotic symptoms in patients with schizophrenia in remission.

Cannabis use and affective disorders

Studies have found mixed relationships between cannabis use and depression. Kandel's early cross-sectional study found that cannabis use was associated with lower life satisfaction and with having consulted a mental health professional or been hospitalized for a psychiatric disorder (Kandel, 1984). Longitudinal analyses of this cohort found weaker associations between adolescent drug use and adult mental health problems (Kandel *et al.*, 1986). Newcomb and Bentler (1988) found strong relationships between adolescent drug use and emotional distress in adolescence, but there were no relationships between adolescent drug use and emotional distress, depression, and lack of a life purpose in young adulthood.

Fergusson and Horwood (1997) found a dose-response relationship between frequency of cannabis use by age 16 and a DSM-IV anxiety and depressive disorder but these relationships were no longer statistically significant after adjusting for confounding factors. Brook *et al.* (1998) reported that early cannabis use did not predict an increased risk of anxiety and affective disorders in young adulthood. McGee *et al.* (2000) reported much the same in a longitudinal study of cannabis use and mental health in a New Zealand birth cohort. Cannabis use at age 15 did not predict mental health problems at age 18.

A number of studies have found associations between adolescent cannabis use and depression. A survey of a representative sample of Australians aged 13–17 years found that those who had used cannabis were three times more likely than those who had never used cannabis to meet criteria for depression (Rey et al., 2002). Fergusson and Horwood (1997) found that 36% of adolescents who had used cannabis 10 or more times by the age of 15–16 years met criteria for a mood disorder at that age, compared with only 11% of those who had never used cannabis. Similarly, the Zurich cohort study of young people followed from 20 to 30 years of age found that by age 30 years, those who had ever met criteria for depression were 2.3 times more likely to report weekly cannabis use (Angst, 1996). A study by Patton and colleagues (2002) of a cohort of young adults (aged 20–21 years) in Victoria found that 68% of females who reported daily cannabis use in the past year were depressed.

A meta-analysis of these studies by Moore et al. (2007) found an association between cannabis use and depressive disorders that was similar to the relationship between cannabis use and psychosis (OR = 1.49 [95% CI: 1.15, 1.94]). They argued, however, that the studies of depression and anxiety disorders had not been as well controlled for potential confounders. Nor had they convincingly excluded the possibility that young people who are depressed are more likely to use cannabis to medicate depressed feelings. They did not rule out the possibility of a relationship, because many of these studies were too small to detect any effect of cannabis use on depression and anxiety disorders.

Henquet et al. (2006) reported a three-year longitudinal study of the relationship between self-reported cannabis use and symptoms of mania in the NEMESIS community sample of 4,848 people in the Netherlands. Their findings on mania substantially replicated their results on schizophrenia. First, cannabis use at baseline predicted an increased risk of manic symptoms during the follow-up period in individuals who had not reported symptoms at baseline. Secondly, there was a dose-response relationship between frequency of cannabis use at baseline and risk of manic symptoms during the follow-up. Thirdly, these relationships persisted when they statistically controlled for the effects of personal characteristics and other drug use.

Suicide

A small number of studies have found a relationship between cannabis use and suicide among adolescents (see Hillman et al., 2000 for a review), but it remains unclear whether this is explained by other risk factors. In the US National Comorbidity Survey there was an association between self-reported suicide attempts and the dependence on alcohol, sedatives, stimulants, cannabis, and inhalants (Borges et al., 2000). The risk for cannabis dependence was still significant after adjusting for socio-demographic factors and other psychiatric disorders (OR of 2.4). Beautrais *et al.* (1999) reported a case-control study of drug use in serious suicide attempts that resulted in hospitalization. They found that 16% of the 302 suicide attempters had a cannabis use disorder (cannabis abuse or dependence), compared with 2% of the 1,028 controls from the community. Controlling for social disadvantage and depression or alcohol dependence substantially reduced but did not eliminate the association (OR of 2).

The evidence from a small number of prospective studies is more mixed. Fergusson and Horwood (1997) also found a dose-response relationship between frequency of cannabis use by age 16 and the likelihood of reporting a suicide attempt, but the association did not persist after controlling for con-founding factors. Patton *et al.* (1997) found that cannabis was associated with self-harmful behaviour among females but not males, after controlling for depression and alcohol use. Andréasson and Allebeck (1990) reported in their follow up of 50,465 Swedish conscripts that the risk of suicide was four times higher among heavy cannabis users.

Moore *et al.*'s (2007) meta-analysis of longitudinal studies of the effects of cannabis use reported that studies of suicide were too heterogeneous to allow combination into an overall estimate of risk. The Odds Ratios (OR) in these five studies varied from a high of 4.6 to a low of 0.6. Few of them were able to exclude reverse causation or properly control for confounding variables, and the one study that had controlled for plausible confounders found that the relationship was no longer significant after statistical adjustment.

The effects of increased THC in cannabis products

Since the early 1970s concerns have been recurrently expressed that cannabis products are becoming more potent (and therefore more harmful to health) than was previously the case (Hall & Swift, 2000; McLaren *et al.*, 2008). Regular monitoring of cannabis products in the United States indicates that THC content has increased from less than 2% in 1980 to 4.5% in 1997 (ElSohly *et al.*, 2000) and more recently to 8.5% (ElSohly, 2008; ONDCP, 2007; see also Chapter 3). THC content also increased in the Netherlands between 2000 and 2005 (Pijlman *et al.*, 2005), and may also have increased in other European countries – although it is uncertain by how much in the absence of time series data on THC in representative samples of cannabis products (EMCDDA, 2004a). Increases in potency have probably resulted from a combination of selective breeding of higher potency plants and a shift to indoor cultivation using the sinsemilla method. All of these trends have been encouraged by the illegal status of the product, which favours the production of more concentrated forms.

The effect of any increase in the potency of cannabis products on health will depend on the extent to which users are able to offset the effects of increased THC by titrating the dose of THC that they obtain (Hall & Swift, 2000). One can conjecture about some of the possible effects of increased cannabis potency. Among naive users, higher THC content may increase the likelihood of adverse psychological effects, such as anxiety, depression, and psychotic symptoms. These may discourage first-time users from continuing to use the drug. Among continued users, increased potency might increase the risk of dependence. If regular users fail to fully compensate for increased potency by titrating their dose, this would increase the risk of psychotic symptoms in vulnerable users. Increased potency could also plausibly increase the risk of road traffic crashes if users do not titrate and drive while intoxicated. On the other hand, any adverse effects of cannabis smoking on the respiratory and cardiovascular systems may be reduced if regular users are able to titrate to a desired dose of THC.

The increased THC content of cannabis may not be the only relevant consideration; changes in the ratio of THC to cannabidiol (CBD), another constituent in cannabis, may also be important. Potter *et al.* (2008) found that cannabis grown using the sinsemilla method has the highest THC:CBD ratio and cannabis resin the lowest. Given suggestive evidence that CBD has anxiolytic and anti-psychotic properties (Morgan & Curran, 2008), research needs to investigate the effect that changes in the THC:CBD ratio have had on the risk of adverse psychological effects from using cannabis.

The adverse effects of cannabis compared to other drugs

Comparisons of cannabis with other drugs

How do these potential harms compare with those of other psychoactive substances in non-medical use?

One important dimension of dangerousness or harm is the likelihood of a fatal overdose (See column 1 of Table 2.1) (Gable, 2004). The 'safety ratio' is the ratio between 'the usual effective dose for non-medical purposes' and the usual lethal dose. Cannabis was in the lowest risk group on this scale, along with other substances that have a ratio of 100 or higher.

Another dimension of dangerousness is the level of intoxication produced by the substance. This is influenced by the dose used, and the set and setting in which it is consumed. Nonetheless, there are differences in the propensity of different psychoactive substances to intoxicate users. The second column of Table 2.1 shows rankings made by Henningfield and Benowitz on this

Table 2.1 Ratings on dimensions of danger

	Safety ratio (Gable, 2004)	Intoxicating effect (Hilts, 1994)	Dependence (how hard to quit) (Hilts, 1994)	Potential addictiveness (Strategy Unit, 2005)	Degree of psychic dependence (Roques, 1999)
Cannabis	>1000 sm	4th highest	Lowest	**	Weak
MDMA	16 or	Nr	Nr	**	?
Stimulants	10 or	Nr	Nr	***	Middling
Tobacco	Nr	5th highest	Highest	***	Very strong
Alcohol	10 or	Highest	4th highest	***	Very strong
Cocaine	15 in	3rd highest	3rd highest	***	Strong but intermittent
Heroin	6 iv	2nd highest	2nd highest	*****	Very strong

Note: Nr = not rated; sm = smoked; or = oral; in = intranasal; iv = intravenous

Safety ratio = (usual effective dose for nonmedical purposes)/(usual lethal dose).

dimension (Hilts, 1994). Cannabis was ranked as more intoxicating than tobacco, but less so than alcohol, cocaine and heroin.

Ratings of the dependence potential or addictiveness of different substances (e.g. Hilts, 1994) compare drugs on withdrawal, tolerance, reinforcement, and dependence. The report of the UK Prime Minister's Strategy Unit (2005) rated drugs on their 'potential addictiveness' and a French committee chaired by Bernard Roques (1999) rated them on 'psychic dependence' (see last three columns of Table 2.1). Although there is some disagreement in the rankings for other drugs, each placed cannabis at the lowest level for the substances in the table.

The Roques committee took a more global approach to rating dangerousness. Table 2.2 shows the committee's rankings on 'Toxicité générale' (general toxicity) and 'Dangerosité sociale' (social dangerousness). In the Roques report, 'toxicity' included long-term health effects such as cancer and liver disease, infections, other consequences of use, and acute effects represented by the safety ratio. The concept of social dangerousness focused on 'states of comportment which can generate very aggressive and uncontrolled conduct … induced by the product or varied disorders (fights, robberies, crimes …) in order to obtain it and risks for the user or others, for example, in the case of driving a vehicle' (Roques, 1999: 296; original in French). The Roques ratings on general toxicity are compatible with the safety ratios of Gable (2004), and the social dangerousness ratings are similar to Henningfield and Benowitz's ratings of intoxicating effect (Hilts, 1994). Cannabis is ranked 'weak' on general toxicity, and 'very weak' on social dangerousness.

Table 2.2 Ratings on global dimensions of dangerousness (Roques, 1999)

	General toxicity	Social dangerousness
Cannabis	Very weak	Weak
Benzodiazepines (Valium)	Very weak	Weak (except when driving)
MDMA/Ecstasy	Possibly very strong	Weak (?)
Stimulants	Strong	Weak (possible exceptions)
Tobacco	Very strong	None
Alcohol	Strong	Strong
Cocaine	Strong	Very strong
Heroin	Strong (except therapeutic use of opiates)	Very strong

Hall *et al.* (1999) compared four substances on whether there was 'important effect' or a 'less common or less well-established effect' on each of 11 dimensions (Table 2.3). According to these rankings, alcohol clearly has the greatest potential for harm while cannabis had the lowest number of asterisks among the four substances rated.

Nutt *et al.* (2007) used the ratings of experts to arrive at a global rating of the comparative harm of different drugs. They identified three main factors that determined the harms of different drugs: (i) the physical harm to the

Table 2.3 Summary of adverse effects on health for heavy users of the most harmful common form of each of four drugs (Hall *et al.*, 1999)

	Cannabis	Tobacco	Heroin	Alcohol
Traffic and other accidents	*		*	**
Violence and suicide				**
Overdose death			**	*
HIV and liver infections			**	*
Liver cirrhosis				**
Heart disease		**		*
Respiratory diseases	*	**		
Cancers	*	**		*
Mental illness	*			**
Dependence/Addiction	**	**	**	**
Lasting effects on the foetus	*	*	*	**

Note: ** = important effect; * = less common or less well-established effect.

individual user; (ii) the tendency of the drug to induce dependence; and (iii) the effect of drug use on families, communities, and society. Within these categories, they recognized three components, to create a 9-category 'matrix of harm'.

Physical harms were split into 'acute', 'chronic', and 'intravenous' harm. Dependence was split into 'intensity of pleasure', 'psychological dependence' and 'physical dependence'. Social harms were split into 'intoxication', 'other social harms' and 'health care costs'. Expert panels of psychiatrists, pharmacologists, and addiction specialists were asked to give scores, from zero to three, for each category of harm for 20 different drugs. Cannabis was rated at eleventh most harmful out of 20 substances. Heroin and cocaine were rated the most harmful, while alcohol and tobacco, the benzodiazepines and amphetamines were rated more harmful than cannabis. Cannabis was scored well below the midpoint of scores on most dimensions. It scored above the midpoint only on intensity of pleasure, intoxication, and chronic physical harm.

The public health impact of cannabis use

Comparisons of the public health burden of cannabis with those of alcohol, tobacco, and other illicit drugs have rarely been attempted because of a dearth of evidence on impact on mortality and morbidity (Hall *et al.*, 2008 in press; Hall *et al.*, 2006). One of the earliest attempts (Hall, 1995) made a qualitative assessment that identified the most important public health impacts of cannabis use 'in order of approximate public health importance' as: motor vehicle accidents; cannabis dependence; respiratory disease; precipitation and exacerbation of schizophrenia in vulnerable individuals; low birth weight babies; and subtle cognitive impairment.

The most recent estimate of the contribution of illicit drugs to the global burden of disease (BOD) confined itself to estimating the contribution of illicit opioid use, because these drugs had the best epidemiological evidence of adverse impact on mortality. Studies estimating the economic costs of alcohol, tobacco, and illicit drugs have often not disaggregated the effects of cannabis from those of opioids (e.g. Collins & Lapsley, 2007). One recent study that did disaggregate cannabis (Rehm *et al.*, 2007) only counted morbidity that could be directly attributed to cannabis via a diagnostic code, namely, episodes of hospital care for cannabis dependence.

A recent Australian study did make a more serious attempt to estimate the contribution that cannabis use made to the BOD in Australia (Begg *et al.*, 2007). This study included estimates of disability due to cannabis dependence and cannabis-related psychoses, and it also attributed small proportions of

MVA deaths and low birth weight infants to cannabis use. It estimated that cannabis was responsible for 0.2% of total disease burden. This comprised 10% of the BOD attributable to the use of all illicit drugs (2.0%), which was a similar proportion to that due to alcohol (2.3%) but a small fraction of that due to tobacco use (7.8%). Even allowing for under-estimation, the contribution of cannabis to BOD on current patterns of use was very modest in a country with one of the highest prevalences worldwide of cannabis use in the late 1990s (UNODC, 2006).

Summary

The acute adverse effects of cannabis use include anxiety and panic, especially in naive users, and an increased risk of accident if a person drives a motor vehicle while intoxicated with cannabis. Women who smoke during pregnancy increase their risk of giving birth to a low-birth weight baby.

The most probable adverse health effects of chronic cannabis use are increased risks of: a cannabis dependence syndrome; chronic bronchitis and impaired respiratory function in regular smokers; increased risk of cardiovascular disease in older adults who continue to smoke into middle age; respiratory cancers in very long-term daily smokers; and psychotic symptoms and disorders in heavy users – especially those with a pre-existing history of such symptoms, a family history of such disorders, or who begin use in their early teens. Among the most *probable* adverse psychosocial effects among adolescents who initiate early are an increased risk of cannabis dependence and impaired educational attainment. Regular adolescent cannabis users have a higher risk of using other illicit drugs, although the explanation of this relationship and its implications remain contentious.

The public health impact of contemporary patterns of cannabis use are modest by comparison with those of other illicit drugs (such as the opioids) or with alcohol. In the former case this reflects the absence of fatal overdose risk from cannabis. In the latter case, it reflects the much lower risks of death from cannabis – lower risks than from alcohol-impaired driving, fewer adverse effects on health, lower rates of regular use to intoxication for cannabis than for alcohol, and the lower rate of persistence of cannabis use into older adulthood.

Annex to chapter 2

Health advice on cannabis

This book is about issues in cannabis policy, and is not primarily concerned with advice to individuals about their own or others' cannabis use. However, we offer here brief advice about cannabis use in the light of the literatures we have just reviewed.

Anyone who is contemplating using cannabis and who wishes to avoid its most probable acute and chronic adverse health effects should abstain from using the drug. This advice is especially pertinent for persons with any disease or condition (e.g. cardiovascular or respiratory disease, serious mental illness or other types of substance abuse) which increases their vulnerability to its adverse effects.

The following advice could be given to cannabis users who do not intend to stop, but who wish to reduce their risks of experiencing adverse health effects.

+ They should not drive when intoxicated (i.e. within several hours of smoking a 'joint'), and should especially avoid driving after combining alcohol and cannabis use, because their impairments may be additive.

+ They could eliminate the respiratory risks of cannabis use by changing from smoking to the oral route. If they persist in smoking cannabis, they should not use the deep inhalation and breath-holding technique which greatly increases the delivery and retention of particulate matter and tar. It is possible to minimise the harms of smoking by using a vapourizer.

+ Cannabis smokers who do not otherwise use tobacco should avoid mixing tobacco with cannabis when smoking a 'joint', if they wish to avoid developing nicotine dependence and the substantial and well-established adverse health effects of tobacco smoking.

+ Cannabis users could minimize the risks of dependence by reducing their frequency of use to weekly or less often, and by avoiding daily use which carries the highest risk of dependence.

- Evidence is emerging that cannabis with high THC and low CBD levels may carry extra risk of psychological harms. High THC and low CBD levels are most commonly found in the genetically modified and hydroponically grown forms of cannabis ('skunk').
- Pregnant women should not smoke cannabis to avoid reduced birth weight.
- There is a convergence of evidence suggesting that initiating cannabis consumption before the age of 17 significantly increases the likelihood of experiencing adverse effects, both personal and social. Children should therefore be advised of these risks.

Chapter 3

The cannabis prohibition regime: Patterns of use, markets, and policies

This chapter reviews cannabis use and the cannabis market in the current circumstances of an international prohibition regime. Prohibition of an attractive substance creates illegal markets, which have consequences in terms of the contours of production, distribution, and consumption. In the first half of the chapter we examine data on the prevalence of cannabis use, the prices that are charged, and the revenues that are generated. The second half examines the enforcement of prohibitions; how many individuals are charged with various kinds of cannabis offences and what are the consequences of those charges. The emphasis is on the developed world, both because more data are available and because there is evidence that use rates are substantially higher in Western Europe, North America, and Australia than in many poorer countries. The emphasis of the chapter is on the effects of full prohibition. We also cover the recent phenomenon of increasing demand for cannabis treatment, as it provides an important rationale in some countries for the continuation of the complete prohibition regimes. Chapters 4 and 5 take up the issue of how variations in prohibition, such as decriminalization, affect the principal outcomes.

Prevalence

In many, but not all, regions of the world, cannabis is the most commonly used illicit drug. It is both cheap per dose and readily accessible to the general population.

Table 3.1 presents data on cannabis prevalence for a number of countries around the world.[2] There is a problem of comparability, dealt with in footnotes,

---

[2] As this book was being written, a new cross-national study of lifetime prevalence and age of initiation was presented for 17 countries that participated in the World Mental Health Survey (WMHS; Degenhardt *et al.*, 2008). Since methodology in this study was

Table 3.1 Prevalence of past year and lifetime marijuana use, among those aged 15–64, ca. 2005

Country	Last year	Lifetime
France[5]	8.6	30.6
Germany (18–59)[3]	6.9	24.5
Netherlands[5]	5.4	22.6
Sweden (16–64)[6]	2.0	12.0
UK[4]	10.3	29.6
USA[6]	10.3	39.8
Canada[4]	14.1	44.5
Australia[4]	11.3	33.6

Note: [3] 2003, [4] 2004, [5] 2005, [6] 2006
Taken from the most recent household survey for each country.

but the major patterns are clear. In many western nations cannabis use is a normative experience; half or more of 21 year olds born since 1970 have tried the drug at least once. There are, however, a few Western nations in which the same is not true. In the Nordic region (other than Denmark), for example, the rates are much lower; a little more than one fifth (21.4%) of youths aged 20–24 have tried cannabis (Collins *et al.*, 2004).

Rates are higher among males than females in all countries, though the rate differences vary. For example, among 15–39 year olds in Switzerland in 2002, the current prevalence rate (roughly speaking, use in the last twelve months) was 4.5% for females and 10.4% for males; the male rate was 2.3 times that of the female. In Canada in 2004, the female rate for those 15 and older was 10.2%, compared to 18.2% for males (Adlaf *et al.*, 2005); the male rate was only 1.8 times that of the female.

Data for non-western countries are much sparser,[3] but suggest more variation across countries and lower rates. For Brazil, a 2005 survey of some

more uniform than in any previous comparison of cannabis use across countries, it would appear to be the most authoritative source for such statements. However, there are large discrepancies between the findings reported in Degenhardt *et al.* and other well-known surveys; for example, for 15–16 year olds in the Netherlands, ESPAD reports a lifetime prevalence rate of 28% while the WMHS shows only 7% for 15 year olds. Consequently, we have not made use of the WMHS data until these discrepancies, which may represent important methodological differences, are accounted for.

[3] The UNODC offers data on regional prevalence rates, but the underlying data sources are opaque, and in some cases it is clear that no systematic data collection underlies the estimate.

metropolitan areas found a lifetime rate for 15–64 year olds of only 6.9% (past year rate 2.6%; UNODC, 2005). Though cannabis has a long history of use in India, often for ritual and religious purposes, a 2001 survey found a past-month rate among males to be 3.0%; the authors of the survey believed that female use rates were very much lower, producing a modest total population rate. China is another major country in which the available data suggest that the drug is of minor importance (UNODC, 2005: 277). There is no tradition of cannabis use in China, where opium was historically the drug of mass consumption. Though the rate in Colombia, an exporter to the US market, is comparable to Western levels (6% in the past year, ages 12–60) (Perez-Gomez, 2005), Mexico, which is the principal foreign producer for the US market, still has low rates: 1.7% lifetime use among adults in Mexico City (Vega et al., 2002).

More data, and more comparable data, are available on use among adolescents as the result of a survey of students aged 15–16 that is carried out every four years in 35 European countries (the European School Project on Alcohol and Drugs survey; ESPAD). The data in Table 3.2 make three points.

Table 3.2 Lifetime drug use among 15–16 year olds in 12 European countries and the United States (2003)

	Cannabis, % used	Cannabis, mean times per student	Cannabis, mean times per user	Any other illicit drug %
Czech Republic	44	7.3	16.6	11
France	38	7.3	19.2	7
Germany	27	4.4	16.3	10
Italy	27	4.9	18.1	8
Netherlands	28	5.0	17.9	6
Poland	18	2.2	12.2	7
Russia	22	2.1	9.5	4
Spain	36	–	–	9
Sweden	7	0.2	2.9	3
Switzerland	40	8.4	21.0	6
Turkey	4	0.6	15.0	3
United Kingdom	38	7.6	20.0	9
USA	36	7.5	20.8	20

Source: European School Project on Alcohol and Drugs (ESPAD) – Hibell et al., 2004.
US rates from Johnston et al. 2007 for 10th graders.

First, cannabis use begins early in many countries; over a third of 15–16 year olds have tried cannabis in 6 of the 13 countries; in only 3 countries have less than 1 in 5 tried the drug. Second, there is substantial variation across countries; even among the wealthier Western European nations, Sweden's prevalence is one-fifth those of many other nations in that group (and the rates in Norway and Finland are similar to those in Sweden). The transitional nations of Eastern Europe already show high rates of cannabis use. Third, there is less variation in the intensity of use, compared to prevalence, by this age group. Almost all nations show an average number of times used of between 10 and 20.

Figure 3.1 presents data on prevalence among younger users in Oslo and the United States, among the few jurisdictions for which consistent data are available over a long period of time. The age groups represented are not identical; 15–20 for Oslo and about 17–18 for the United States; but the purpose is not to compare absolute rates but rather changes over time. The two series differed in the 1980s, with the US youth rate declining sharply while that for Oslo was stable. However since the early 1990s the two series have been very parallel, rising through most of the 1990s and declining modestly since then. Similar trends for the period since 1990 can be found in less complete data in other countries such as Australia and the Netherlands.

Though cannabis initiation does not show the same strikingly short epidemics as cocaine and heroin in Western countries (see e.g. Nordt & Stohler, 2006), there have been periods of nearly explosive growth and of smaller but still sharp declines. For example, the prevalence of cannabis use (last 12 months among those aged 15–64) in France rose by 150% between 1992 and 2002 (UNODC, 2008: 115), while in Australia the prevalence (last 12 months among those aged 14 and over) fell by nearly 50% in the period 1998–2007 (UNODC, 2008: 118).

Duration and intensity

Prevalence of use is only part of the story. Equally important are the duration of cannabis using careers and the intensity of use during those careers. A few studies show that the majority of users use the drug only a few times but that many do have careers of regular, if not frequent, use that extend for over 10 years. For example, Perkonnig et al. (2008) studied a cohort in Munich aged 14–24 at first interview in 1995–1998. By final interview in 2005, over half the sample reported at least one incident of cannabis use. Most relevant here is that 40% of those who reported using cannabis at their initial interview, when interviewed 10 years later, reported using the drug in the previous 12 months. The rate was, as might be expected, particularly high among those who had used five or more times at the baseline interview.

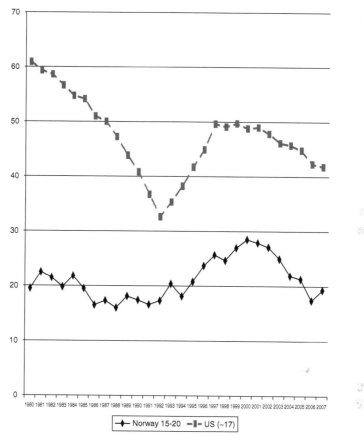

Fig. 3.1 Percent youth reporting ever used cannabis, Oslo and the United States, 1980–2007.
Sources: US data from Monitoring the Future; Norway data from Bryhni, 2007.

The one published long-term study of a cohort of American youth shows long periods of daily cannabis use (defined as 20 days in the previous month) for a large proportion of the sample. Kandel and Davies (1992) report on a cohort of 10th and 11th graders recruited from New York State high schools in 1971. When the respondents were re-interviewed in 1984, at age 28 or 29, over one quarter (26.2%) had been daily users of cannabis for at least some one-month period in their life. Even more striking, the mean duration of spells of near-daily use was over three and a half years. The much greater involvement

Table 3.3 Intensity of use by frequency of use by males

# of joints per consumption day	12 to 30 days per year	31 to 54 days per year	55 to 234 days per year	235 to 365 days per year
1	70.2%	58.8%	41.6%	31.6%
2	18.7%	25.8%	26.9%	27.2%
3	6.6%	5.7%	10.7%	21.3%
4	1.3%	2.8%	4.6%	3.7%
5	2.4%	3.2%	4.4%	4.3%
6 or more	0.8%	3.8%	11.9%	11.9%

Source: National Household Survey on Drug Abuse (1991–1993)
Public Use Data Files: http://webapp.icpsr.umich.edu/cocoon/SAMHDA-SERIES/00064.xml
Prepared by Jon Gettman, October 2009
Reformulation of Table originally published in Gettman (2007).

of this sample in cannabis use may be cohort- and location-specific;[4] this was a group which went through the high risk years near the peak of the counter-culture movement, and many were from New York City, which was particularly influenced by that movement.

The figures on intensity of use are striking. The EMCDDA (2004) thought that it was reasonable to assume that 1% of the population aged 15–64 used cannabis on a daily basis. Large numbers use multiple times per day. Analysis of 2001 Australian survey data suggest that those who use daily or nearly daily consume on average about four joints per day (Pudney *et al.*, 2006; 67). During the period 1991–1993 the National Household Survey on Drug Abuse (NHSDA) in the United States collected detailed data on frequency of use. Of those males who used most days of the year, about 40% used three or more joints per day on days that they used (Table 3.3).

This very skewed intensity of use distribution is similar to that typically found for alcohol; in surveys of alcohol use, the heaviest 20% of US drinkers account for 87–89% of total consumption (Greenfield & Rogers, 1999). Efforts to estimate the same parameters for cocaine and heroin using general population surveys are unpersuasive, since those surveys are known to omit the majority of frequent users of these drugs; indeed in the United Kingdom,

---

4 This is consistent with national data. For example, in the Kandel and Davies study over 70% reported use at some time prior to the interview. The closest comparison is with the 1979 NHSDA 18–25 year olds – that is, those born between 1956 and 1961. This comparison is appropriate because most initiation occurs before age 20. The NHSDA figure for lifetime use of marijuana was 68%; no data are available on the two-year birth cohort of 1955–1956.

United States, and many other countries, no effort is made to provide estimates of the extent of dependent or heavy use of heroin from household surveys. Thus we cannot compare the skewness of use patterns for cannabis with those for cocaine or heroin.

In many surveys, relatively few of those who tried cannabis have experienced problems as a consequence. However, a major survey focused on such matters; the National Comorbidity Survey in the United States found that about 10% of users responded in ways which qualified them for a dependence diagnosis at some stage in their life (Anthony *et al.* 1995), a matter we take up more fully later. Few go on to use more dangerous illicit drugs; the 1995 US National Household Survey on Drug Abuse found that only 23% of 26–34 year olds who had used marijuana[5] at some time had also used cocaine during their lives. Moreover, that fraction has declined in the United States for more recent birth cohorts (Golub & Johnson, 2001).

Summary

Despite its prohibition in every country apart from the Netherlands, experimentation with cannabis is a routine experience among adolescents in many Western nations. Use is more common among males than females, but even among females a large proportion has tried the drug by their early adult years. A substantial fraction of those who experiment go on to use the drug frequently, and a modest share of those experience problems of dependence. The rates of experimentation vary considerably across countries at the same level of economic development, probably reflecting broad cultural and social factors.

Price

The price of cannabis plays two roles in our analysis. On the one hand it is a measure of the effectiveness of the control regime, because prohibition aims to make the drug expensive and difficult to obtain. A modest body of research consistently demonstrates that cannabis consumption (as measured by prevalence) is responsive to price (see Grossman, 2005 for a review). Higher price, *ceteris paribus*, will lessen prevalence and consumption, for an illicit good as for a licit one.

The second role of price is as one determinant of dealer revenues. If the price of marijuana were comparable to that of cigarettes, before taxes, then one important adverse consequence of marijuana prohibition would be eliminated,

---

[5] Since cannabis herbal resin is almost unknown in the United States, we generally refer to marijuana rather than cannabis in citing US figures.

namely the corruption, violence, and diversion of labour that it now generates, since the potential revenues for individual dealers would be modest. While it is strictly speaking profits rather than prices that determine the attractiveness of the trade, data on profits do not exist; moreover, in terms of the incentives for stealing drugs (a potentially major source of violence), it is their value, not profit margins, which matter.

Price data for illegal drugs are always weak, reflecting the difficulty of developing a good sampling frame and sampling strategy for illicit markets. For cannabis there is an extra problem, which is a lack of data on potency. It is plausible that more potent marijuana, precisely because it has more of the active ingredient, will be more expensive per gram, but perhaps no more expensive per unit of THC. The Dutch data on price and potency are roughly consistent with this latter hypothesis (Pijlman *et al.*, 2005).

Potency

A standard claim is that prohibition leads to production of more potent forms of a substance, since higher potency reduces the bulk and hence the risk associated with distribution. There is evidence for this with respect to alcohol during American Prohibition, during which the illicit market for alcohol became almost entirely spirits (Warburton, 1932). The same was true for opiates in Thailand in the 1980s (McCoy, 1991). For cannabis, any such effect has certainly been slow to manifest itself. The potency of cannabis remained quite low relative to what was technically attainable until the 1990s, 25 years after the emergence of major markets in a number of Western nations.

It is known that the THC content of cannabis varies substantially across countries and time periods; it may be as low as 2% or as high as 20%. A recent survey of potency in Europe (EMCDDA, 2004) found that potency had not consistently increased in recent years, and that in most countries it remained in the range of 6–8%. The Netherlands was an exception, with potency having risen from already high levels to figures that were never considered before, close to 20% (Niesink *et al.*, 2005), see Fig. 3.2. Unfortunately the only data set that consistently records potency in connection with price is that from the Netherlands, which covers purchases in coffee shops where the drug is *de facto* legal.

In general, there is reason to believe that average potency has increased over time in many countries. Less authoritative data are available over a longer period for the United States.[6] They also show a large and sustained increase

----

6 These data come from seizures of marijuana primarily though not exclusively from federal agencies. If law enforcement authorities are more likely to seize imported than the

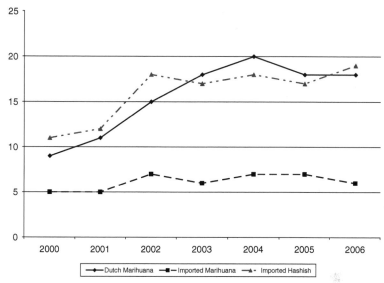

Fig. 3.2 Average THC percentage in cannabis products, the Netherlands, 2000–2006. Source: Niesink *et al.*, 2005.

in the potency, from around 3% in the mid-1980s to about 9% 20 years later (Fig. 3.3).

Variations in potency mean that the various price series below may not correctly measure effective price, and comparisons across countries are particularly perilous.

Price

As usual, more price data are available for the United States than for any other country. Figure 3.4 (from Caulkins *et al.*, 2004) shows retail and wholesale prices (at two levels) for marijuana from 1981 to 2003.[7] Taken at face value (i.e. ignoring unmeasured changes in potency), this suggests that prices rose during the 1980s, declined during the 1990s, and rose again in the first half of this decade. Caulkins (1999) has shown that this variation in prices can indeed

----

domestically produced drug, then they will probably underestimate the potency, since the domestic is more likely to have been grown with high potency. An increase in the share that is domestically produced will tend to lead to an increase in the difference between the market average and the average recorded in the test data.

[7] The data are from System to Retrieve Information from Drug Evidence (STRIDE), which includes data on all seizures and purchases of drugs by federal agencies and from a few state and local agencies. For a discussion of the strengths and weaknesses of STRIDE see Caulkins (2001) and Horowitz (2001).

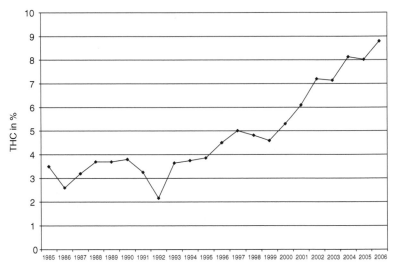

Fig. 3.3 Average marijuana potency, seized material, USA.
Source: The University of Mississippi Cannabis Potency Monitoring Project, quoted in US Department of Justice, National Drug Intelligence Center, 2008.

account for most of the observed fluctuation in last-year marijuana use among high-school seniors up to 1998; prevalence declined during the 1980s and rose during the 1990s. The data from the government potency monitoring study suggest that marijuana potency has been increasing sharply at least since 1990 (see Fig. 3.3), so price trends may be misleading.

For other countries, cannabis price information is scarce. For example, Pudney (2004: 437), in a careful analysis of cannabis use in the United Kingdom, noted that 'The only systematic source of price information comes from the National Criminal Intelligence Service (NCIS). This goes back no further than 1988 and gives only *ad hoc* ranges of street prices reported by police drug squads in various locations.' The EMCDDA published in 2005 estimates of cannabis prices for a number of its member states. The underlying data are of varying quality; some may be little more than police guesswork. Table 3.4 presents these figures, along with data for the United States, Canada, and Australia.

The EMCDDA (2007c) reported that, adjusted for inflation, cannabis prices had fallen in all but one of the countries reporting data. One of the few other analyses of prices over time is that of Clements (2004), using data for Australia; he found that over the 1990s, the real price fell by 40%.

It is useful to compare the price of cannabis to that of other sources of intoxication. In the United States a standard drink (e.g. a 12 oz. can of inexpensive beer)

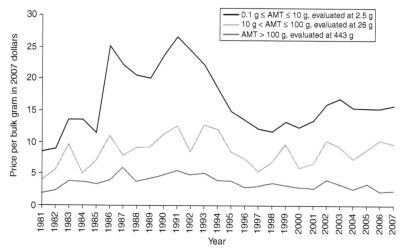

Fig. 3.4 Price of 1 g of marijuana, United States 1981–2007.
Source: Office of National Drug Control Policy, 2008.

costs about $1, at package store (off-sale) prices. For the average person, a moderate level of intoxication would require about three drinks. If a joint contains 0.4 g, at a price of $12 per gram, it only costs $5 to get high. The comparison is of course a very rough one, but it indicates that prohibition still leaves cannabis competitive with a taxed legal commodity as a source of intoxication.

Table 3.4 Price of cannabis circa 2005 (in US dollars)

Country	Price per gram
France	5.60
Germany	6.57
Italy	6.41
Netherlands	5.28
Spain	3.47
Sweden	8.49
Switzerland	6.18
UK	3.36
Canada	8.10
US	12.30
Australia	15.26

Sources: EMCDDA, Caulkins *et al.* (2005).

Quantities and expenditures

A nation's cannabis problem is not measured merely by the numbers of users but also by the quantity consumed and the amount of money spent. Most harms experienced by users are an increasing function of the quantity consumed; if each gram of cannabis used increases the risk of a driving accident, then it is useful to estimate the total quantity consumed. Expenditures represent the size of the black market available for bribes to officials, and the temptations to youth to divert labour from legitimate activities. Unfortunately, there are few estimates of either quantities or expenditures.

The best documented estimate is for the United Kingdom, developed by Pudney *et al.* (2006). Like all such estimates, it relies on self-reports of use and intensity of use and must therefore be regarded as a lower bound figure. Even with alcohol it has been impossible with self-report population surveys to replicate total consumption and expenditure estimates based on tax records; developing an estimate as high as two-thirds of the known figure has been about the best any scholar has been able to attain (Greenfield *et al.*, forthcoming). Pudney *et al.* estimate that in 2003–2004 total cannabis consumption in the United Kingdom was about 400 tons and expenditures totalled £1 billion; this compared to £40.8 billion for alcohol and £15.6 billion for tobacco in 2004 (Harris, 2005: 246).

Table 3.5 presents the few national estimates of cannabis consumption and expenditures per capita for recent years, along with expenditures per user and as a share of GDP. If the underlying surveys are as accurate as those for alcohol, which seems optimistic, the quantity estimates should be increased by 50% to provide a more realistic figure. Nonetheless, it remains the case that cannabis expenditures are small compared to those for alcohol and tobacco.

Kilmer and Pacula (2009) have re-estimated cannabis revenues for a number of Western countries. Combining these with the UNODC (2005) estimates for other markets (accounting for only 22% of the UNODC global estimates), they calculate the total retail sales for cannabis worldwide to be only $40–$80 billion in 2005, compared to the UNODC estimate of a total of $142 billion for 2003. The international trade value may be very low because so much of what is consumed in Western countries is now produced domestically.

The markets for cannabis

Estimates of cannabis production

Cannabis differs from the other major natural base illegal drugs, cocaine and heroin, in that it is produced in many of the major wealthy consumer countries.

Table 3.5 Marijuana consumption and expenditures: Existing estimates of the retail market for cannabis

Country	Source	Year	Amount (metric tons)	Nominal value	2005 Euros (billions)	% GDP
Australia	Clements & Zhao, 2005	1998	339	AU$ 5.35 B	4.14	0.90%
Finland	Hakkarainen et al., 2007	2004	1.7–4.3	–	–	–
France	Legleye et al., 2008	2005	–	€ 746–832 M	0.75–0.83	0.05%
NZ(1)	Wilkins et al., 2002	1998	–	NZ$ 131–170 M	0.09–0.11	0.15%
NZ(2)	Wilkins et al., 2005	2001	–	NZ$ 190 M (131–249 M)	0.12	0.16%
UK(1)	Bramley-Harker, 2001	1998	486	GBP 1.58 B	2.55	0.29%
UK(2)	Pudney et al., 2006	2003–2004	412 ±155	GBP 1.031 B ±0.433 B	1.55	0.19%
US (1)	ABT, 2001	2000	1,047	US$ 10.5 B	9.92	0.10%
US (2)	DEA, unpublished	2000	4,270	–	–	–
US (3)	Drug Availability Steering Committee, 2002	2001	10,000–24,000	–		–
US (4)	Gettman, 2007	2005	9,830	US$ 113 B	99.97	0.91%
World (1)	UNDCP, 1997	1995	–	US$ 75 B	80.10	0.25%
World (2)	UNODC, 2005	2003	35,663	US$ 142 B	125.6	0.38%

Notes: Based on estimates of availability, not necessarily consumption (e.g. some could be exported or confiscated by local authorities). Estimates not directly comparable because of different populations and methods. Nominal values are inflated using the CPI published by the OECD and then converted to Euros using the conversion rate for 1 July 2005 from xe.com/ict. GDP figures were obtained from EconStats.com. Data for US(3) publicly available at: http://www.whitehousedrugpolicy.gov/publications/drugfact/drug_avail/
Source: Kilmer & Pacula, 2009.

One hundred and thirty-four countries reported cannabis production in their territory, according to the UNODC (2007). Most produce only for domestic consumption. This makes it particularly difficult to estimate the total production of cannabis (Leggett & Pietschmann, 2008), since it is not produced in large fields in concentrated areas of a few countries; the latter characteristics have simplified the task of estimating global opium and coca production.[8] Leggett and Pietschmann (2008) discuss the official global estimates of about 40,000 tons with appropriate caution. It is hard to reconcile that figure with an estimated consumer population of 160 million. If we use 100 g as a relatively generous estimate of the per user annual consumption; this yields a total quantity less than half as big (160 million × 1/10 kg = 16,000 metric tones). Seizures in 2006 amounted to about 7,000 tons, according to the *2008 World Drug Report*; seizures were concentrated in Mexico and the United States.

Not much is known about markets for cannabis, but at least three characteristics come through from the existing literature in a number of countries:

1 Very large numbers of persons are involved in distributing the drug, and large numbers in growing it. Gettman (2007), analysing data from the US National Survey on Drug Use and Health, reports that almost 2% of respondents reported that they had sold an illegal drug in the previous 12 months; among respondents aged 18–24, the figure is 6%. This covers all drugs, not just cannabis, but it is likely that the vast majority are involved in cannabis selling. A forthcoming paper by Bouchard *et al.* (in press) reports data from a school in a part of Quebec province that is known to have high involvement in cannabis production. Bouchard *et al.* found that 15% of youth reported being involved in growing cannabis.

2 Imports from the developing world account for a modest and decreasing share of the rich world's consumption. The Netherlands estimates that the domestic production from approximately 18,000 'cannabis farms' was between 130 and 300 tons of cannabis in the early part of this decade (van der Heiden, 2007). This was far more than might be consumed by Dutch users and the coffee shop visitors (less than 80 tons). Some of this is exported to other Western European nations. Bouchard (2008) estimates that production in the province of Quebec in 2004 totalled 300 tons, of which less than one-third was consumed in the province. Most of the rest was presumably shipped across the land border with the United States.

---

[8] For a discussion of the absurdity of earlier US estimates of Mexico's marijuana production, see Reuter (1995).

As a corollary, the length of the distribution chain for cannabis is much shorter than those for cocaine or heroin. For example, it is quite plausible that heroin passes through an average of ten transactions between the poppy farmer and the final customer (Paoli *et al.*, 2009). Although there are occasional border seizures of multi-ton shipments, it is clear that much of the cannabis is delivered through chains with no more than two or three links between the producer (a local grower) and the end user.

3 Violence is not commonly found in cannabis markets. This is mostly an inference from the absence of reports rather than any positive information that disputes between market participants are resolved amicably and that competition for territory is lacking. The United States always figures prominently in accounts of violence in drug markets. Even though cannabis involves many more producers, sellers, and dealers than cocaine or heroin, there are only occasional references to homicides or other kinds of violence in the market. A recent investigative report of the grey market in 'medical marijuana' in California remarked on seeing 'thousands of Tibetan prayer flags' along the way, which served to 'identify their owners with serenity and the conscious path, rather than with the sinister world of urban dope dealers, who flaunt muscles and guns' (Samuels, 2008). Gamella and Jimenez Rodrigo (2008) report some incidents of violence in the upper levels of the import trade in Europe, but also comment that the violence seems substantially less than that involved in markets for cocaine or heroin. Korf *et al.* (2008), reporting on a sample of youth sellers of cannabis in four countries, find only 10% who had been assaulted or injured in the course of this business, much less than the rate for youth selling other types of drugs.

Cannabis, more than other illegal drugs, seems to be acquired within social networks, with purely market transactions as a secondary source of acquisition. Caulkins and Pacula (2006) analysed the National Survey on Drug Use and Health and found that most users reported that they acquired their marijuana from a friend (89%) and for free (58%). There certainly are street markets of the conventional variety, but this is not, at least in the United States, the principal mode of acquiring the drug. Caulkins and Pacula estimate that in 2001 there were about 400 million purchases, each involving an average of marijuana equivalent to about 7 joints. This estimate is broadly consistent with 2 million sellers, most of them very much part-time dealers, who make 200 sales per annum and have gross revenues of about $5,000 each. The fact that the market is so imbedded in social networks may be an important factor in explaining the lack of violence.

Production for own use is a substantial source of cannabis in some countries. For example, Atha *et al.* (1999) estimated that 30% of cannabis consumed in the United Kingdom was home grown, while in New Zealand a majority of respondents reported that at least some of what they consumed was home grown (Wilkins *et al.*, 2002). Analysis of US survey data also shows that much is given away; Caulkins and Pacula (2006) found that 58% of users reported that the marijuana acquired most recently was given to them free.[9] In Spain, Gamella and Jiménez Rodriguez (2004) report a number of indicators of increasing home cultivation since 1992, in response to a change in Spanish law that allowed the police to make a criminal arrest for transporting cannabis.

Unsurprisingly, young people in many Western countries report that the drug is readily available to them. Even in the ESPAD survey of 15–16 year olds, as many as 80% of respondents in some European countries report that they can obtain cannabis. In the United States, the percentage of high-school seniors reporting that marijuana is available or readily available has been over 80% for the last 30 years.

Summary

Though cannabis is very much more expensive than it would be if it could be legally produced and remained untaxed, the drug is readily available in many Western societies at a cost that allows cannabis to compete with alcohol as a source of intoxication. This is partly explained by the fact that it can so readily be produced within rich countries in small quantities that are often traded within social networks. Nonetheless, the cannabis trade totals tens of billions of dollars globally.

Cannabis policies

With few exceptions, most countries are signatories to the international conventions (see Chapter 6) requiring the prohibition of cannabis production, sale, and possession, with criminal penalties. Famously, the Dutch do not enforce the prohibition in certain circumstances, but the law on the books does specify possible criminal penalties even for possession. Various other jurisdictions, as discussed in Chapter 4, have decriminalized possession to a greater or lesser extent by way of changes to the law, but all retain a prohibition on the commercial production and sale of cannabis.

----

[9] As might have been expected, it was those who used less frequently that were most likely to have received the drug for free. A far smaller share of the quantity consumed was given away free.

With these interesting exceptions applying to a tiny fraction of the population of the developed world (analysed in detail in Chapters 4 and 5), the important variation in the nature of national cannabis use control is determined by how the law is administered. It is a tale about practical law enforcement, pure and simple.

We give no discussion of source country control programmes, a staple of efforts to reduce cocaine and heroin consumption. Although Mexico and Morocco are important suppliers of cannabis products to the United States and European markets respectively, they account for a modest share of the total market, and there is little faith that eradication of their production would have much impact on its availability. Another difference is that seizures of cannabis, although they constitute two-thirds of all drug seizures and are even substantial as a share of total cannabis consumption (perhaps as much as one-third), get little attention as a policy tool.

Arrest for use or possession

Cannabis arrests account for the majority of drug law arrests in most Western countries. For example, in Australia they accounted for about three quarters of all drug arrests in the period 1995–2000, while in Germany in 2005 they accounted for 60% of the total; cannabis possession and use offenses alone were 45% of the total.

Figure 3.5 presents some data on cannabis arrest rates per capita in a number of Western nations around 2005. Switzerland stands out in this respect with over 600 arrests per hundred thousand population. The United States has a rate of about 300 per hundred thousand, not much more than various other Western European nations or Australia. These arrest figures are a mix of formal arrests and citations. In some countries even a citation will be recorded as an arrest, but in others that is not the case. In some countries the rates include only arrests for which the cannabis offence is the most serious offence; in others it includes all offences in which cannabis is included.

In many countries, cannabis arrests have risen sharply since the mid-1990s. For example, in Switzerland cannabis arrests totalled about 17,000 in 1997 (15,500 for consumption) and had risen to over 29,000 (26,000 for consumption) by 2002; that figure has since declined slightly. In the United States there was a massive increase in cannabis possession arrests starting in 1991. The number more than doubled in three years (226,000 in 1991 to 505,000 in 1995) and has continued to rise sharply, so that by 2006 it was estimated to be over 735,000, a 45% increase in 11 years. Australia is unusual in that it has seen a decline of one-third over the period 1995–2005.

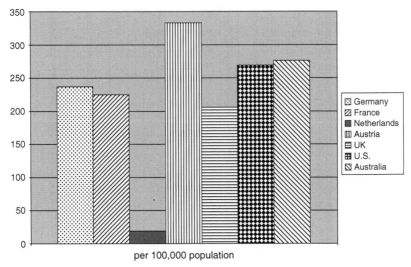

Fig. 3.5 Arrest rates for cannabis possession per 100,000 population, ca. 2005.

Arrest rates per capita of course vary a great deal by age and sex and, where the data are available, by race. In Australia, males are arrested four times as frequently as females. In Switzerland the ratio is over five to one. These are much higher than the male–female ratios of prevalence of use cited earlier, but they have not been adjusted for intensity of use, so that the risk per use occasion may not differ much between the sexes.

The age gradient can be very steep. Table 3.6 shows the rates for cannabis possession arrests in five-year age groups in the State of Maryland, USA, in 2000. The rate among 15–19 year olds is almost nine times the rate among those aged 35–39. The same pattern can be seen in data from Switzerland. In 2002, the arrest rate for cannabis possession for males aged 18–24 was about

Table 3.6 Cannabis possession arrest rates per 100,000 in different age groups, Maryland, 2002

Age range	Arrest rates per 100,000
15–19	1657
20–24	1410
25–29	563
30–34	249
35–39	193

Source: Reuter *et al.*, 2001.

4,000 per 100,000, twice the rate for those aged 25–34, and over six times the rate (600) for those aged 35–49.

Data by minority status specific to cannabis are hard to find outside the United States. In the state of Maryland in the period 1980–1997, the ratio of rates for whites and African-Americans have varied substantially; the rates were about equal in the early 1990s, but by 1997 the rates for African-American residents were twice as high as for white residents.

To some extent the arrest rate reflects differences in cannabis use prevalence by group. Males have higher use rates than females and use is most common among those aged roughly 16–24. However, when one adjusts for differences in prevalence by age, it still appears that younger users are at substantially higher risk of being arrested than are their older counterparts. This may reflect the relative indiscretion of youthful users and the fact that they spend more time in exposed settings and have less opportunity for use in private places than older adults. Studies of arrests for smoking marijuana in a public place in New York City, where the arrests fall disproportionately on blacks and Hispanics (Golub *et al.* 2007), found that observing 'etiquette' about not smoking in public, etc. made a difference in the likelihood of arrest in poor black neighbourhoods, but not elsewhere (Johnson *et al.*, 2007).

Punishment for use or possession

Arrest of course is just the first step in the criminal justice process. It is just as important to have data on the steps and punishments that follow arrest. In general the data show that, for cannabis possession or use, punishments other than fines are rare. For example, Lenton *et al.* (1996) report that in Western Australia in 1993, well before it decriminalized the offence of cannabis possession, 94% of arrestees (including those charged with possession of paraphernalia) received a simple fine and only 0.3% received a custodial sentence. Weatherburn and Jones (2001) report that in the Australian state of New South Wales in 1999, just 1.2% of those convicted of cannabis possession or use were sentenced to prison, and such punishments typically came when the cannabis use offence happened in conjunction with other offences and/or the offender had an extensive criminal record. In Switzerland, the vast majority of cannabis possession offences result in a fine of less than 250 Swiss Francs (about $250 in 2008), and are not recorded as convictions in aggregate statistics.

In the United States, data on dispositions of cannabis arrests are hard to find precisely because they are prosecuted as misdemeanours and most data systems are set up to track the disposition of more serious offenses (felonies). Golub *et al.* (2006) report that in New York City marijuana possession arrestees 'face a day in jail pending arraignment (if detained) … and the remote possibility of a few additional days in jail if convicted' (p. 133). Reuter *et al.* (2001) studied the disposition of arrests for simple possession of marijuana in three large counties in one state (Maryland) that has not decriminalized drug use but is generally seen as liberal in its policies. The study found that almost no arrestee received a jail term as a sentence, but that one in three of all arrestees spent at least one night in jail and one out of ten spent at least ten nights in jail.

There are, however, more subtle effects that should not be ignored. Imposing a criminal conviction can create barriers to employment in some occupations and organizations and lead to loss of other privileges (see Chapter 5). Thus, for instance, a criminal conviction may lead to rejection of an application for a US visa. This and more proximal adverse social impacts of criminal conviction were significant considerations in the Western Australian parliament moving minor cannabis offences to a non-criminal category.

Risks to dealers or growers

In contrast to users, those arrested for smuggling, growing, or dealing can face serious punishment. Even the Netherlands, with its tolerant policy towards cannabis consumption, is aggressive in its pursuit of growers and traffickers. Korf (2008) reports that the number of prosecutions for cannabis growing rose from 4,324 in 2000 to 6,156 in 2003 (about 4 per 10,000 population). Switzerland, another country with a well-established reputation for liberal drug policies, also prosecutes relatively large numbers for marijuana dealing or growing, with nearly 4,000 individuals in 2003, or 8 per 10,000 population. On a *per capita* basis these figures may be close to that for the United States.[10] For Europe as a whole, there appear to be no data on incarceration specifically for cannabis production or distribution offences.

In the United States, the penalties for dealing or growing can be very severe indeed; Schlosser (1994) discusses some egregious cases, in which an individual engaged in marijuana growing received a sentence of over 20 years. In the federal courts, which generally only handle cases involving large quantities of the drug, nearly 6,000 individuals were convicted of cannabis offences in 2007, mostly for selling and importing; 97% pled guilty, and the average sentence length was just over three years (Sourcebook of Criminal Justice Statistics, 2007, Table 5.25.2007). Interestingly, 41% of those sentenced were foreign born, compared to just under 30% for federal drug offenders in general (Table 5.39.2007). This suggests how much the high-level trade involves natives of

---

[10] No data exist in the United States for prosecutions by drug type. The statement is simply an informed judgment.

other countries, even if they may be more likely to be caught than US citizens.

How tough is enforcement or how risky is use?

Cannabis is a mass market drug. Very large numbers of arrests may still mean that any individual user is at quite low risk of being apprehended. For example, Weatherburn and Jones (2001) estimated that in New South Wales, Australia, with 7,820 arrests for cannabis in 1999 (approximately 122 per hundred thousand population), only one in approximately 100 marijuana users appeared in court charged with this offence, and that fewer than one in 10,000 of a prison-eligible age were sent to jail for the offence.[11]

Table 3.7 provides rough estimates of user risk of arrest annually for seven nations around 2005.[12] In no country was the rate more than 5%. Indeed, the narrow range for all these countries, except the Netherlands with its official tolerance, is surprising given the formal differences between countries where police have discretion about whether to make an arrest and others, such as Germany, in which the police are required to respond to any violation they observe.

Another way of performing the risk calculation is to estimate the probability that any given occasion of cannabis use results in arrest. The intensity of cannabis use is, as already noted, quite variable over the current user population. However a substantial fraction or users use it more than once per week. For example, in Finland Hakkarainen et al. (2008) estimated that about 5% of users consumed daily, and an additional 15% consumed weekly but less frequently than daily. The total of 106,000 users consumed about 3 tons (averaging the high and low estimates), with each joint containing an average of 0.4 g of cannabis; this yields 7.5 million joints or about 75 joints per user per year. If each joint represented a separate use event, the probability of detection for any given joint then becomes vanishingly small, less than one in one thousand.

---

[11] Weatherburn and Jones do the calculations of rates for those who were arrested for cannabis possession only; these constitute about 40% of all arrests involving the charge of cannabis possession. The figures reported here include the larger population of arrests.

[12] The comparisons are even rougher than they look because in some countries what is counted is the number of unique individuals arrested each year, while in others it is the number of unique arrest events. The latter may include some individuals who have been arrested previously in the same year. We think this makes only a modest difference to what is at best an indicative rather than precise measure.

Table 3.7 Cannabis arrest rates for 7 countries, ca. 2005

	Per 100,000 population	Per 1000 users*
Germany	237	34
France	225	26
Netherlands	19	3
Austria	333	44
United Kingdom	206	20
United States	269	31
Australia	276	24

*Users: estimated number of past year users from most current household survey.

The calculation is different, and even more speculative, if we inquire as to the risk of a user getting caught in the course of a cannabis use career. We suggest a simple approach. Estimate the probability of arrest per consumption episode and then assign each user the average number of consumption episodes per annum over the average number of years. If there is a one in 3,000 chance of being arrested for any one episode and the average career involves 300 use episodes, then a user has a one in ten chance of being arrested at some stage. A more sophisticated version of this categorizes users by intensity of use and calculates the probability for each category.

The reason for conducting this 'career risk' calculation is that the decision made by a user can be modelled on the assumption that the user is either myopic or far-sighted. This has been the center of the contentious debate about 'rational addiction', the model that Gary Becker and Kevin Murphy (1988) developed for the study of the demand for addictive substances. In our adaptation of the model, the myopic user considers only the risk of being arrested for his first use; the far-sighted (perhaps 'rational') user takes into account the risk over his expected lifetime of use. Given that user careers begin in early teenage years in many countries, the myopic model is more appealing, but it is worth knowing the likelihood of arrest in the course of a user's entire career.

The calculation here is highly speculative because there is a great deal of heterogeneity both in arrest risks and in number of episodes. However using crude averages for the United States, we calculate that a user has a 30% chance of being arrested in the course of a career that is on average 10 years long. The calculation should be refined before being taken seriously.

What are the consequences of tougher enforcement?

On its face, enforcement of cannabis prohibition seems unsuccessful. Certainly it has not succeeded in preventing cannabis use becoming a routine behaviour for a large percentage of young people in many Western countries. Although the actual punishments imposed are quite modest, it is reasonable to ask whether the large numbers of arrests have a deterrent effect.

This turns out to be a difficult question to answer for methodological reasons. The relevant measure of intensity of enforcement is the probability of arrest conditional on use; however that means that the percentage of the population using cannabis appears in the denominator on the right hand side of the equation, as well as in the dependent variable, creating potential bias.[13] Cross-national studies are unlikely to be persuasive, since there are many other factors that affect prevalence which cannot readily be specified. Within-country studies have more plausibility, but they require a measure of cannabis use at the subnational level to match with enforcement intensity. There are few countries with a federal structure that allow such analysis.

Pacula *et al.* (2003) use marijuana arrest rates per capita and marijuana arrests as a share of all police arrests in modelling differences in prevalence of use among youth across US states. They find that neither arrests variable is significant, replicating the results of a similar model, with different data, by Farrelly *et al.* (1999). The literature is thin, but provides no evidence that higher rates of arrest are associated with lower rates of cannabis use.

Treatment-seeking by cannabis users

A relatively new phenomenon is large-scale treatment-seeking by cannabis users. In many Western countries there has been a rapid and sustained increase in the number of treatment admissions for which cannabis is identified as the principal drug of abuse. For a recent review of the treatment literature, see Bergmark (2008), who finds evidence that many modalities have substantial beneficial effects on cannabis use and related problems, but that no modality seems superior to others. Our purpose here is to document the rise in the flow of clients and to assess what drives it.

The EMCDDA (2007a), on the basis of data from 21 of its 25 member countries, estimated that cannabis was the primary drug of abuse for 20% of all treatment cases in EU countries in the most recent year for which data were available. Even more strikingly, in 2005 the share of all first admissions to

---

[13] Another potential problem is that prevalence of use may influence the state's decision about how many arrests to make, just as arrests may influence prevalence.

treatment accounted for by cannabis was 29%. The total number had trebled between 1999 and 2005. Cannabis admissions were exceeded only by those for heroin. The rates and rates of increase varied considerably across countries within Europe; for France cannabis admissions were 30% of all treatment admissions, whereas for some other EU countries the figure was less than 5%.[14]

In the United States the increase had begun earlier but was similarly startling in magnitude, given that overall cannabis prevalence had remained quite stable since 1988. Whereas in 1992 cannabis was the primary drug of abuse for 10.2% of all admissions, that percentage had risen to 15.8% by 2005; the total number of cannabis admissions was 171,000 in 1992 and 292,000 in 2005. In the latter year, cannabis was the most frequently cited primary drug of abuse among admissions.

In Canada, a study of Ontario treatment admissions in 2000 found that cannabis was the drug most frequently cited as the primary cause for admission (Urbanoski et al., 2005). A later study of admissions to publicly supported treatment programmes between 2001 and 2004 found that about one quarter of all admissions reported cannabis problems (Rush & Urbanoski, 2005).

Even with this increase, the share of all cannabis users in treatment programmes at any one time is very small. For example, the EMCDDA estimates that past year users totalled 23 million in 2004; treatment admissions totalled about 65,000, barely three-tenths of 1% of the total. The figure looks slightly different if one makes the assumption that all those seeking treatment are frequent users (which is questionable to the extent that some are referrals from the criminal justice system).[15] The EMCDDA estimate of daily users in the European Union is 3 million. If all those in treatment were daily users, this would suggest that about 2% of daily users were receiving treatment. This is well below the corresponding figure for heroin, which is as high as 50% in some EU countries.

Another way of looking at the figures is to compare the annual numbers of new daily users and of new treatment admissions. If the system were in steady state, which it is not, this would provide a rough estimate of the probability

---

[14] The comparisons offered here are only for the longer term EU countries (the 15 members in 2004, before additional members were admitted), since most of the new members were still in transition in terms of drug use prevalence.

[15] Montanari et al. (2008) report that the data on frequency of use among those seeking treatment appears to be quite poor. Nearly 30% report either no use or infrequent use in the month before admission, which is an unlikely figure except perhaps for criminal-justice referrals.

that a daily user receives at least one episode of treatment. Unfortunately there are no systematic estimates of the number of new daily users, so one can make only rough back-of-the-envelope calculations. If time spent in the state of being a daily user is 20 years, then there might be 150,000 new daily users in Europe; the new treatment admission figure of 40,000 would then look very high. We offer this merely as a very speculative basis for suggesting that in the future treatment may become a common experience for those with cannabis dependence problems.

What has driven this increase in treatment seeking? Certainly many factors are potentially involved and their importance varies across countries:

Prevalence. In some countries treatment demand may simply track increased use. That clearly is implausible for countries such as the United Kingdom, the Netherlands, or the United States, where total population prevalence is either flat or declining.

Intensity of use may have increased, as measured for instance by the share of all past-year users who used daily, indicating that a higher fraction of users have problems. In Europe, only recently have national surveys included detailed data about frequency of use, so that in general there is not trend data for this part of the problem. For the United States, the National Survey on Drug Use and Health (covering the years 2002–2004) for the age group 18–25 found that 4.3% were daily users of marijuana in the previous year, constituting 15% of past year users in that age group.

Criminal justice referrals. For the United States, the rapid rise in arrests for marijuana possession is certainly a factor. One method of minimizing the chance of a serious sanction for such an arrest is to be able to inform the judge that the defendant is in a drug-treatment programme. A high fraction of those classified as marijuana treatment admissions in 2005 (58%) were listed as criminal justice referrals, much higher than the fraction for either cocaine or heroin (SAMHSA, 2007). However, given that there are almost no arrests for cannabis possession in the Netherlands, that is unlikely to be a factor in the increase in that country. There may also be forms of 'soft coercion' from schools and teachers that also play an increasing role.

Supply of treatment places. Only recently have treatment providers begun to offer specialized services for cannabis users. This may be an independent influence; treatment providers may be responding to the decline in demand for services specific to other drugs, in countries such as the Netherlands with an ageing and slowly declining population of dependent heroin users.

Awareness of potential harms of frequent cannabis use. There has been increasing media coverage of the possibility that cannabis use might lead to schizophrenia or psychosis. This may have caused more users with careers of frequent use to seek to stop and, in face of problems in doing so, to seek therapeutic help to accomplish that goal.

The list can be easily lengthened. For example, higher potency might cause more problems, improved record-keeping might mean that a higher percentage of actual cases are captured in statistics, while declining age of first use might lead to earlier identification of problems by users. There may have been shifts in the settings in which the drug is consumed that have increased harms. No doubt still others will emerge with further research.

Under a system of prohibition that has not changed much in the past decade, there has been a sudden surge in the numbers seeking help in dealing with problems associated with cannabis use. The increase has been observed in many nations with long histories of cannabis use. The numbers are now large enough in many countries to suggest that cannabis use is a significant problem for at least a modest proportion of all users and a substantial proportion of heavy users. For our purposes the treatment seeking increase is a reminder that the problems associated with a drug are determined by many factors and are not a timeless constant, a point that is well understood in the alcohol policy field. For example, changes in patterns of drinking can have profound effects on the adverse consequences of a given per capita alcohol consumption. The same may be true for cannabis, and the appropriateness of a particular policy will depend on that.

The current status

As will be described in Chapter 4, there have been moves to a less punitive regime in a number of countries. In the election of November 2008, for instance, voters in the US state of Massachusetts voted by a 65% majority to reduce the penalty for possession of less than an ounce of marijuana to a civil fine of $100 (Abel, 2008). But the prohibition regime is not at immediate risk, and there are also some steps in the opposite direction. For example, in 2008 the British government, with Prime Minister Gordon Brown leading the way, and against the advice of the official expert advisory committee, moved to increase the severity of penalties for drug possession and sale,[16] reversing an easing of penalties that occurred in 2004. The maximum penalty for supplying is to be raised to 14 years, and possession penalties to a maximum of five years. The rationale for this change, to be achieved primarily through the revision

---

[16] The Home Office announcement of the change in policy can be found at http://www.homeoffice.gov.uk/drugs/drugs-law/cannabis-reclassification/

of the scheduling of cannabis from Class C to Class B, is primarily the new evidence discussed in Chapter 2 of an association between cannabis use and psychosis, particularly schizophrenia.

The event serves as a useful reminder that efforts to reverse cannabis prohibition or to substantially lessen the severity of the regime can readily be reversed. Popular support for cannabis prohibition is surprisingly strong. Eurobarometer, the principal survey of opinion in the European Union, reports that only about one quarter of respondents favoured the legalization of simple possession of cannabis. Support for major changes in the legal status of marijuana possession laws has also been low in the United States for the 30-odd years that the Gallup poll has asked the question. This provides a base of support for increasing the severity of penalties when perceptions of the potential dangers of the drug increase.

As discussed, however, there is minimal evidence that changes in statutory penalties would reduce cannabis use. The lack of evidence of a deterrent effect has to be weighed against the considerable harms that undoubtedly arise from the existing regime. Cannabis is a drug used by very large proportions of the populations of many Western countries. There is a large-scale black market that is an unintended consequence of the existing system of prohibition, as acknowledged recently in an essay by the Executive Director of the United Nations Office on Drugs and Crime (Costa, 2008). The cannabis market causes less harm than similarly sized black markets for cocaine and heroin since it is associated with less violence and probably less corruption; the latter is a consequence of the more dispersed production and shorter distribution chains. Nonetheless, a global black market of tens of billions of dollars represents in itself a challenge to the authority of governments. While there is little systematic study of harm at institutional or societal levels specifically from cannabis markets, there is no doubt that the existence of large illicit markets tends to foster organized crime, and corruption of police and of political institutions. A few studies suggest that Brazil is one country in which the industry is concentrated and organized enough that it has generated high levels of at least regional violence and exploitation (e.g. Iulianelli *et al.*, 2004; Zaluar, n.d.). But there is a dearth of documentation of broader harms to producer societies.

The arrests of many hundreds of thousands of cannabis users in the Western world might also be called a harm. That might not be the case if arrest were typically the prelude to provision of treatment, as is increasingly the case for heroin in some countries such as the United Kingdom, and if those arrested were likely to be users with treatable problems. However, there is nothing about the arrest process that suggests that it targets high-rate and problematic users; instead, it seems that arrestees are users who are unable to act discreetly or who simply are unlucky. A modest percentage of arrestees are referred to treatment. Thus, unless there is evidence of deterrent effect, arrest in itself seems to cause harm to some users without many compensating benefits. We note, though, that in most countries there is little formal punishment beyond the arrest itself. It is, accordingly, important not to exaggerate the severity of the harms suffered by arrested users.

Finally, there must be a nagging concern about the fairness with which cannabis laws are enforced. The small amount of available evidence suggests that police often use the charge of cannabis possession as an easy way of harassing or making life difficult for marginalized populations. It is often an excuse for intrusion into their lives, allowing a search which might turn up something else of interest for the police.

In the following two chapters, we turn to the various efforts and experiments which have been made at national or subnational levels to ameliorate these harms, considering first the nature and scope of the efforts, and then the evidence on their effects.

Chapter 4

The range of reforms within the system: Softening the prohibition

Introduction

Background

This chapter reviews the existing reform models of cannabis control that have been implemented at national and subnational levels around the world within the provisions of the existing international treaties and conventions. It describes the control regimes which have departed from a standard approach of full criminal prohibition, and reviews the evidence of the impact of these alternative regimes on cannabis use and other indicators. Before examining the details of the reform regimes, we clarify: the wider social, legal, and practical context; how the alternative regimes have evolved; and the key concepts, terminology, and typologies used.

While prohibitions of, or controls on cannabis began in some places in the early decades of the twentieth century, cannabis was not formally integrated into international drug control efforts until the 'International Opium Convention' adopted in 1925 in Geneva (Mills, 2003; Rödner-Sznitman *et al.*, 2008; Zeese, 1999). Following the Convention's provisions, nonmedical cannabis use became subject to criminal controls in nations subscribing to the Geneva Convention and its successor agreements. This included making illegal not only to produce, distribute, and sell cannabis, but also to purchase, possess, and use the drug, after 1961 even for medical use. Thus Article 33 of the 1961 Single Convention on Narcotic Drugs provides that 'the parties shall not permit possession' of cannabis 'except under legal authority', and Article 36 enjoins each party, 'subject to its constitutional limitations', to make cultivation, transport, sale, purchase, or possession 'punishable offences when committed intentionally'. Since this wording was still seen as providing too much leeway for national variations, Article 3 of the 1988 Convention, without any allowance for constitutional limitations, specified that such acts should be established 'as criminal offences under domestic law'.

Cannabis became the main target of drug enforcement in many Western countries in the 1960s when, for example, the number of arrests for drug offenses in countries such as the United States or Canada increased to unprecedented levels due to massive increases in arrests for cannabis use (Bonnie & Whitebread, 1974; Giffen *et al.*, 1991; Slaughter, 1988). Arrests for possession or use figured prominently among the arrests. As a consequence, large numbers of predominantly young people were receiving criminal convictions, fines, and in some cases, custodial sentences. This, in turn, triggered considerable social debate around the appropriateness of criminal cannabis use control in several countries in the latter half of the 1960s. One feature of this debate was a number of large-scale public inquiries or commissions over the following decade, with committees in Australia ('Senate Social Committee on Social Welfare', 1977), Britain ('Report by the Advisory Committee on Drugs Dependence', 1969), Canada (Commission of Inquiry into the Non-medical Use of Drugs, 1973), the Netherlands (Baan and Hulsman Commissions, 1970 & 1971), and the United States ('Shafer Commission', 1973) reporting between the late 1960s and late 1970s (UKCIA, 2000). Most of these inquiries concluded in essence that many of the harms perceived for cannabis use were exaggerated, that the effects of the criminalization of cannabis use were potentially excessive and the measures even counterproductive, and that lawmakers should drastically reduce or eliminate criminal penalties for personal use of cannabis. However, in most jurisdictions – the Netherlands probably being the notable exception (Cohen, 1997) – these recommendations for cannabis law reform did not result in substantive policy reform in the short term.

Over the past couple of decades or so, however, several Western jurisdictions have seen changes to or reforms in the ways cannabis use is being controlled, departing from traditional approaches of criminal prohibition that have dominated cannabis use control regimes on national levels for most of the twentieth century. Well-known earlier examples of such reforms include the Netherlands and several US states, where distinct changes to cannabis use control towards less punitive interventions were first implemented in the late 1970s (EMCDDA European Monitoring Centre for Drugs and Drug Addiction, 2007b; MacCoun & Reuter, 1997; Single, 1989). More recently, reforms have been implemented or proposed in an increasing number of countries, including countries of the European Union, Australia, or North/Central America. Most of these changes have been assessed by expert commentators to be occurring within the bounds, that is, within the parameters and requirements, set by the international drug control treaties as applicable to cannabis use control on national levels (e.g. Krajewski, 1999), although this point can be contested.

Conceptual issues, terminology, and typologies of reform

The alternative cannabis use control regimes that have evolved in different jurisdictions in recent years are characterized by considerable heterogeneity in their key characteristics. This complexity makes their analytical examination challenging. As in any analysis of law enforcement, one critical difficulty is that there are numerous discrepancies between the 'law on the books' and the 'law in action'. In other words, the law has a 'social dimension', and the 'making of crime' is a process influenced by subjective factors (Boyd, 1986; Chambliss, 1975; Ericson & Baranek, 1982). Concretely, the enforcement of existing law – especially based on the power of discretion given to the various institutions of the criminal justice system, notably the police – often occurs selectively or arbitrarily, or even under dynamics of systematic bias (Beckett et al., 2006; Kellough & Wortley, 2002; Weitzer & Tuch, 1999). For example, considering cannabis use enforcement specifically, local police in a city may actively enforce standing law against many, only some, or no cannabis users, while practices elsewhere in the same country may be entirely different, or change from time to time. Such inconsistencies in enforcement can result from local or regional variations in enforcement practice, from the involvement of different levels of legislative or enforcement jurisdictions (e.g. the co-existence of federal, state, and local law and police in the United States), and from variations in enforcement priorities across time and place, or from differential approaches to perceived situational and individual offender characteristics (Bayley, 1994; Smith & Visher, 1981). Furthermore, both the prosecution and key agents of jurisprudence (e.g., judges) in democratic systems of law have considerable discretion in their decision-making once a charge has been laid (Gottfredson, 1987; Kessler & Piehl, 1998). For example, the prosecution can decide not to prosecute a charge; the courts can decide to acquit the offender, or to impose any of a wide range of sentences (e.g. probation, community or intermediate sentence, fine, jail time) allowed by the applicable statute. These variables make existing cannabis use control provisions and practices a complex and often inconsistent area for examination.

One important analytic distinction between different types of alternative cannabis use control regimes is thus the differentiation between *de jure* and *de facto* reforms. The former refers to reforms that are written into and stipulated by the letter of the law, while the latter are realized by the way the law is used or applied in the various stages of the criminal justice system (Fischer et al., 2003; McDonald et al., 1994).

The longstanding debate around cannabis use control – in the wider context of drug law and policy reform – has included a number of terms which have not always been consistently applied or clear in their meaning. In general, *criminal control or criminal sanctions* refer to when cannabis use is defined as a criminal offence by a statute enshrined in criminal law, a criminal charge (e.g. a felony or a misdemeanour charge in the US system) is brought, and a public record ('criminal record') is kept following a conviction in court (Hall & Pacula, 2003). The confusion arises in the terms used for measures which in one way or another move away from full criminal sanctions – '*decriminalization*', '*depenalization*', and '*legalization*'. In this chapter, we follow Pacula *et al.* (2005) by using the term 'depenalization' to refer to any change of cannabis use control provisions in the letter or practice of the law that *reduces the severity of the penalties* – whether criminal or civil – imposed on the offender. The label of 'depenalization' therefore could include reforms that retain the criminal status of cannabis possession as an offence, yet remove or shorten the periods of incarceration, or reduce fine amounts, as possible sanctions. The term 'decriminalization', then, will be used only to refer to reforms which change the status of cannabis use *from a criminal to a non-criminal* (e.g. a civil) offence. Thus, reform measures of 'decriminalization' can be viewed as usually a sub-category of 'depenalization', although it can be that the civil penalties are more onerous than the criminal. Since 'decriminalization' in turn has often been misunderstood, the term 'prohibition with civil penalties' has been seen as preferable to 'decriminalization'. The removal of all punitive sanctions from cannabis use is often described as 'legalization'. However, federal alcohol Prohibition in the United States never included criminalization of possession or use of alcohol, and it is not usually thought of as a 'legalization' regime. Furthermore, it is likely that even if cannabis sale were legalized it would still be governed by different tools of regulatory law (e.g. public health, commercial, or workplace laws).

Several observers have offered analytical frameworks for classifying cannabis use control reforms as they have occurred in different jurisdictions (Fischer *et al.*, 2001; Hall & Pacula, 2003; McDonald *et al.*, 1994; Pacula *et al.*, 2005). There is considerable overlap between the different typologies, though they are useful tools to order and analytically examine the increasing number and variety of reform measures. In this chapter, our examination of cannabis use control reform builds on the typologies originally presented by McDonald *et al.* (McDonald *et al.*, 1994). Our analysis is thus structured around the following regime categories:

- Full prohibition (i.e. no reform)
- Prohibition with cautioning or diversion ('depenalization')
- Prohibition with civil penalties ('decriminalization')

- Partial prohibition, including:
  a) '*De facto* legalization' (e.g. prohibition with an expediency principle)
  b) '*De jure*' legalization
- Medical marijuana control

Table 4.1 lays out some comparisons of the characteristics of four of these categories: depenalization, decriminalization, and the two varieties of partial prohibition. In this chapter, we provide exemplary illustrations and descriptions of cannabis use control reform regimes within the different categories as they have been occurring or proposed in different countries. In the following chapter, we turn to the available evidence on the impact of these reforms.

Cannabis use control reform regimes and examples

In this section, we will briefly describe key features of the individual cannabis control reform regimes, and then provide examples and illustrations from jurisdictions in which such models have been implemented. It should be noted here that the list of examples given is selective and not exhaustive, and is mainly from established market economies, reflecting the availability of relevant data and information.

It should be noted that departures from the international prohibition regime, at least *de jure*, have primarily concerned the individual cannabis user. The main aim of the various regimes has been to lessen the burden of criminality on possession and use, and in some places on cultivation for one's own use. Even in the most far-reaching regimes, there is no explicit legalization of production or distribution of cannabis products, which would be contrary to a number of provisions of the international conventions besides those on use and possession.

Depenalization – prohibition with cautioning or diversion

General remarks

Under some cannabis use control regimes that would formally be described as *total prohibition*, with cannabis use formally prohibited and punishable by criminal law, *informal or intermediate justice* measures are applied at various stages of criminal justice processing (Baker & Goh, 2004; Bammer *et al.*, 2002; Erickson & Oscapella, 1999; Lenton *et al.*, 1999). These can include *cautioning* or *diversion* of offenders to alternative measures, including treatment. *Cautioning* is typically applied by law enforcement in pre-arrest situations where an offence (e.g. a cannabis

Table 4.1 Typology of cannabis use control reforms

Reform type	Prohibition with cautioning/ diversion ('depenalization')	Prohibition with civil penalties ('decriminalization')	Partial prohibition ('de facto' legalization)	Partial prohibition ('de jure' legalization)
Modus operandi	Cannabis use is prohibited by criminal law, yet alternative measures (e.g. pre- or post-trial diversion; diversion to treatment) at various stages of the criminal process reduce the severity of punitive consequences.	Cannabis use is illegal, yet controlled by non-criminal statutes or interventions (e.g. administrative/civil law in form of a 'ticketing offense'). Criminal processing and consequences are eliminated.	Cannabis use is formally prohibited by criminal law, yet applicable laws are not enforced or suspended in practice ('de facto') at select stages of the criminal justice system.	Cannabis use is shielded from punitive consequences or explicitly permitted by relevant legal norms (e.g. drug control law).
Comments and concerns	In most instances, the key impacts of criminal prohibition (e.g. criminal conviction/record) remain despite depenalization provisions. Measures may lead to over-use of or inappropriate diversion.	Key negative consequences of criminal punishment are removed, yet possible problem of 'net-widening' and 'secondary criminalization' (e.g. due to fine default) exists.	Normative ambiguity, i.e. discrepancy between 'law on books' and 'law in action'. Situation hinges extensively on discretion of agents of the criminal justice system, and law on books can be selectively enforced.	Such provisions are most likely to be in violation of the international control treaties. Existing 'de jure' legalization provisions mainly aim at select spaces (e.g. the home) or populations (e.g. medicinal marijuana users).
Examples	Several US states; United Kingdom	Several Australian states	The Netherlands, Germany	Alaska; Medical Marijuana provisions in parts of US and Canada

possession offense) is encountered and a formal arrest could be made, yet instead of an arrest, the matter is dealt with by warning or cautioning the offender about his or her behaviour and its possible consequences. *Cautioning* can occur fully *ad hoc* and informally based on law enforcement's discretion in the specific circumstances of a situation, or on the basis of more formalized 'cautioning schemes' that include procedural guidelines on when to apply cautioning. These sometimes involve a written notice and/or record-taking, or possibly imposing an intervention in order to avoid more formal consequences (Macintosh, 2006). In the United Kingdom, for instance, police cautioning is normally predicated on an offence being admitted, and is entered in police records. In its effects, such a procedure can be argued not to differ greatly from plea-bargaining to a lesser criminal charge in the United States.

Diversion measures or schemes are usually more formalized procedures aiming to shift offenders from the criminal justice system and its mainly punitive consequences to education, treatment, or other interventions typically aimed at changing behaviour (Ashworth, 2005; Bull, 2003; Sherman *et al.*, 1998). *Diversion* can occur at various stages in the criminal justice process, including pre-arrest, pre-trial, pre-sentence, or in the actual sentencing based on diversion schemes (Bull, 2005; Lattimore *et al.*, 2003; Passey *et al.*, 2006; Spooner, 2001; Ulrich, 2002).

Pre-trial diversion schemes, which operate in the time after a charge has been brought, but prior to the charge being dealt with in court, usually involve the offender engaging in certain assessment, education, or treatment conditions as part of bail conditions or at the behest of the prosecutor. *Pre-sentence diversion* measures focus on the period after conviction, but prior to sentencing, or utilize diversion measures as an active substitute for conventional sentencing (e.g. fines or time in correctional institutions). These measures can involve the offender being put on remand while he or she attends assessment and treatment, and performance in this is usually taken into account when he or she is eventually sentenced. *Diversion measures at the sentencing stage*, that is, in lieu of conventional sanctions, can occur in the form of community-based or rehabilitation measures (e.g. courses, information sessions, community service) or treatment programmes. In recent years, for example, 'drug treatment courts' (DTCs) or other so-called 'therapeutic justice measures', involving a combination of punitive tools and therapeutic interventions typically over longer periods, have become popular post-charge diversion programs for drug offenders in North America (Belenko, 2001; Goldkamp *et al.*, 2001; Taxman & Bouffard, 2002; Turner *et al.*, 2002). Cautioning or diversion measures have been introduced and increasingly applied in response to frustrations with the limited effects of conventional justice measures. They are also motivated by the desire for more 'constructive' or rehabilitative interventions, limiting the negative effects (e.g. labelling) of criminal justice involvement. They are commonly used for young or first offenders, but may also be available to others, such as repeat offenders. Other factors in promoting cautioning or diversion measures are cost-reduction considerations – cautions consume considerably less police time than arrests, and diversions may reduce expensive court or jail time (Justice Research and Statistics Association, 2000; Shepard & Blackley, 2007).

France

In France, cannabis possession is technically a criminal offense as stipulated by the narcotics control law. Available information suggests however that for personal cannabis possession offenses, 'there might be no further action' (European Legal Database on Drugs, 2004b) in most instances, that is, prosecution is waived in the context of an overall diminishing proportion (e.g. 10%) of cases of illegal drug possession being prosecuted. Furthermore, a range of diversion measures exist for illicit drug users coming into contact with the criminal justice system in France. It is suggested that 'mere drug users are mainly dealt with by therapeutic alternatives' (e.g. by way of a 'therapeutic order') or a request to contact social or health services, and thereby avoid criminal prosecution. Furthermore, a new law from 1999 provides a range of diversion measures for 'certain minor offenses, particularly related to mere drug use', including a voluntary fine payment or community service, in lieu of criminal prosecution (European Legal Database on Drugs, 2004b). It is not clear, however, from the available data to what extent or how systematically these alternatives are applied in cases of personal cannabis possession.

Australia

Four of Australia's eight states and territories (New South Wales, Victoria, Queensland, Tasmania) apply 'prohibition with cautioning' schemes for minor cannabis offenders, with other states applying 'prohibition with civil penalty' schemes (see below) (Baker & Goh, 2004; Hall, 2008; Spooner, 2001). These former – cautioning – schemes are limited to minor possession and implement (bongs, pipes, and other smoking equipment) offences, but not to cultivation of cannabis. To be eligible for a caution the cannabis offender must admit to the offence and agree to attend an education session on cannabis, an assessment session concerning drug use problems, or drug treatment, depending on the jurisdiction. Essentially when the offender agrees to a cautioning notice, prosecution for the offence is suspended for a set period (usually of 2–4 weeks) to allow the person to complete the intervention stipulated by the caution.

Those who fail to successfully complete the requirement are charged with the original offence. Typically, those with a history of violent offences are excluded from the cautioning schemes. Depending on the jurisdiction, cautions may be applied to the first as well as to second or third cannabis offences, but not to subsequent offences, for which criminal sanctions then apply. Possession limits for which cautioning procedures may be used also vary from state to state, ranging from 15–50 g, and may involve an intervention requirement including a mandatory assessment for drug treatment or a brief intervention.

Canada

Cannabis use in Canada is currently controlled formally by a regime of 'full prohibition' in which even small amounts of cannabis possession are followed by a criminal charge and possible penalties (up to a maximum of 6 months in jail and/or $1000 fine for a first offense) under the federal 'Controlled Drugs and Substances Act', CDSA (Fischer *et al.*, 2003; Senate Special Committee on Illegal Drugs, 2002). Over the past decade, the number of arrests for cannabis possession offenses in Canada has roughly doubled, and they now make up about half of all arrests under the CDSA, emphasizing cannabis as the primary target of drug enforcement in Canada (Silver, 2007). However, a couple of relevant reform provisions or efforts concerning cannabis possession control have been introduced in recent years. One of these reforms involves the vehicle of so-called 'Conditional Sentencing' introduced into criminal law provision and practice in Canada in 1996. 'Conditional Sentencing' is a sentencing diversion mechanism creating the possibility for offenders in certain specified offense categories (e.g. non-violent offenses) to be processed by intermediate sentencing following a guilty plea to the original criminal charge and subsequent conviction, and thus to reduce the extent or impact of penal sanction in favour of more rehabilitative measures (Roberts & Cole, 1999). Strictly speaking, 'Conditional Sentencing' measures applied to drug offenses are thus not a measure of decriminalization, yet can result in depenalization effects (e.g. where a drug use offender would receive a treatment or community service order instead of a fine). Since its inception, the application of Conditional Sentencing in Canada has embraced a steadily increasing number of drug offenses, including some cannabis possession offenses, mainly imposing treatment orders in lieu of or in conjunction with other sentencing (Hendrick *et al.*, 2003). Early evaluations show that in Ontario, between 1997 and 2001, the proportion of conditional sentence commencements for drug-related offences more than doubled (Hendrick *et al.*, 2003). Later research illustrates that federally in 2003 drug-related crime (2,518) was the third largest category of convictions, in terms of actual numbers, for which conditional sentencing provisions were used, following property crime (4,215) and various forms of assault (2,565) (Statistics Canada, 2007). Its use, however, depends on discretionary decisions by the court. Unfortunately, no detailed data are available on the exact use, nature, or outcomes of conditional sentencing measures specifically for drug offenders in Canada, and certainly the majority of cannabis possession offenders in Canada are currently being dealt with by standard criminal procedures and sanctions as outlined by the CDSA.

Britain

Pressure for reform of British cannabis laws increased during the 1990s as the public became increasingly tolerant of cannabis use, and law enforcement practice was increasingly making use of 'cautioning' instead of charges following an arrest for cannabis possession (Collison, 1994; Warburton *et al.*, 2005). In 2000, an independent Inquiry into the Misuse of Drugs Act of 1971 recommended that cannabis should be reclassified from a Class B to a Class C drug, resulting in lessened criminal control over personal use and possession of the drug. The reasons given were that cannabis was less harmful to health than most other Class B drugs; and the reclassification, which would make cannabis a non-arrestable offence, would remove the burden of criminalization from a large proportion of young people. Following a further inquiry, advice being sought from the Advisory Council on the Misuse of Drugs and a 'successful' trial of a cannabis pilot scheme utilizing 'informal' warnings – which, in contrast to 'cautioning' procedures, do not result a criminal records entry – for cannabis possession offenders in the London borough of Lambeth in 2001, the British government reclassified cannabis as a Class C drug on 29 January 2004 (Ellison, 2004; Pearson, 2007; Warburton *et al.*, 2005). However, in an apparent attempt to balance calls for reform against increasingly vocal opposition, reclassification was preceded by an amendment to the Police and Criminal Evidence Act (PACE) 1984 making possession of a Class C drug an arrestable offence (May *et al.*, 2007), thus eliminating this key de-penalizing element of the re-classification. Concurrent with reclassification, the London Metropolitan Police issued an operations notice to officers stating that, in cases of cannabis possession for personal use where no aggravating factors were present, based on the officers' discretion the individual should not be arrested. An accompanying Police Standard Operating Procedure postulated a presumption against arrest for adult cannabis possession, with a decision in favour of arrest requiring justification. Further, adults who were arrested could be dealt with by no further action, by cautioning or by a charge as appropriate (Leigh, 2007). The various changes in the legal control of cannabis use in a relatively short period apparently caused some confusion among the British public with regard to the status of the drug, and also considerable inconsistencies among law enforcement practices. A multi-site study comparing the policing of cannabis possession incidents before and after the re-classification found that, while a large minority of cannabis possession incidents in the study sites were disposed of by informal warnings, the majority still involved arrests followed by formal cautioning or charges as the main intervention (see Pearson, 2007; Warburton et al., 2005). Hence, the authors of one study concluded that the reclassification of cannabis has had 'a smaller impact than advocates hoped ... and opponents feared' (Pearson, 2007: 1176). The differences in enforcement practices were found to be associated with both officer and offender characteristics. As noted in Chapter 5, in 2008, against the advice of the Advisory Council on the Misuse of Drugs, the government moved to reclassify cannabis back to Class B.

United States

While overall the United States, through its various layers of drug control laws, is characterized by a full prohibition regime, it is widely documented that 11 US states 'enacted legislation during the 1970s that reduced the criminal sanctions associated with possession of small amounts of marijuana' (Pacula et al., 2003: 4 ; see also Single, 1989). Predominantly, these state laws downgraded the legal status of marijuana possession offences, defining possession of small amounts as a misdemeanour, that is, reducing the severity of penalties following violations while retaining them formally as criminally sanctioned offenses under this offense rubric. Thus, while these reforms have widely been labeled as 'decriminalization', it has been suggested that this may have been a misnomer in strict terms, and these reductions are more appropriately described as 'depenalization' (Pacula et al., 2005). Currently, several US states (e.g. Oregon, Colorado, Ohio, Maine, Minnesota, Mississippi, New York, Nebraska, Connecticut, Louisiana, Massachusetts, New Jersey, Nevada, Vermont, Wisconsin, and West Virginia) – including nine of the original so-called 'decriminalization' states – carry reform legislation depenalizing personal possession of marijuana. However, formally most of these statutes even today do not meet formal 'decriminalization' standards, and furthermore differ in key features. For example, while most US reform states process marijuana possession as a misdemeanour, others have these offenses categorized as a 'civil violation' or a 'petty offense' (National Organization for the Reform of Marijuana Laws (NORML), 2008). Fine amounts for possession offenses vary from state to state (e.g. ranging from $100 to a maximum of $1000 in some states), while in some states jail sentences are possible in theory for repeat or even first offenses. Some of the US states featuring cannabis depenalization regimes also include provisions for diversion measures, for example, probation, community service, drug education programmes, or probation with mandatory treatment (NORML, 2008).

Another approach to depenalization was adopted by popular referendum in California in 2000, under Proposition 36, the Substance Abuse and Crime Prevention Act. While the measure applies to non-violent possession offenses for any drug, some affected cases involve cannabis. The Act permanently changed state law to allow qualifying defendants convicted of non-violent drug possession offenses to receive a probationary sentence in lieu of incarceration (Fratello, 2006). As a condition of probation, defendants are required to participate in and complete a certified drug treatment programme. If the defendant fails to complete the treatment programme or violates other aspects of their probation, probation can be revoked and the offender may be required to serve an additional sentence possibly including incarceration. While some 250,000 drug offenders have been processed under the initiative to date, evaluation data from various years and counties since Proposition 36 was enacted show that offenders with marijuana as their primary drug of offence have consistently been a minority representing approximately 12–14% of offenders (Appel et al., 2004; Fosados et al., 2007; Longshore et al., 2003). Approximately one in three offenders diverted complete their treatment; however, one-third of these completers are re-arrested for another drug offense within one year. It should be noted that Proposition 36 is a post-conviction diversion measure focusing on sentencing measures; it does not eliminate the principal legal status or consequences of a conviction for a cannabis use offense. In cases where incarceration is replaced by treatment – and such treatment is successfully completed – as part of the sentencing imposed for a cannabis use conviction, the severity of punishment imposed is considerably reduced, or a depenalization effect is realized, although this in practice appears to occur only for a minority of offenders included in this programme.

Brazil

In 2006, Brazilian legislation removed the possibility of a jail penalty for possession of drugs. Previously, those caught possessing small amounts of drugs faced between six months and two years in prison, but the new law substituted one or more of the following penalties: treatment, community service, fines, or suspension of the offender's driver's license. In the same law, the minimum penalties for drug traffickers and sellers were increased, and a new crime was created of being a 'narcotrafficking capitalist', punishable by between 8 years and 20 years in prison (Drug War Chronicle, 2006). In March 2008, a Sao Paulo appeals court ruled that Brazil's drug law was unconstitutional with respect to punishing drug possession. It is not yet clear what the effect of this ruling will be (Drug War Chronicle, 2008).

Prohibition with civil penalties (e.g. fines and administrative sanctions)

General remarks

Under this cannabis control reform regime, possession or use remain explicitly outlawed. However, legal control frameworks have been implemented in which specifically defined forms of cannabis possession (typically limited to possession of cannabis for personal use) are exempt or sheltered from criminal control provisions. Instead, a non-criminal punishment (e.g. a civil citation or infringement notice), a monetary penalty (e.g. a limited fine), or some other administrative sanction (e.g. temporary revocation of one's driver's license) is levied, with no further criminal consequences or involvement of the criminal justice system. Activities relating to larger scale possession and production, as well as sale or other supply activities of cannabis, usually remain subject to conventional criminal control procedures and penalties.

Civil penalty schemes aim to reduce the punitive impact (e.g. stigmatization or criminalization) and public costs or resources associated with traditional criminal control of minor cannabis possession (Erickson, 1980; Erickson & Murray, 1986; Lenton & Heale, 2000; Lenton et al., 2000b). This is done while maintaining the illegality of cannabis, to maintain a clear normative stance that cannabis use is wrong and any general deterrence effects against cannabis use, and to arguably remain within the bounds of the international conventions. In systems where small-scale cultivation or purchases of cannabis products for personal use are included in the non-criminal exemptions, the inclusion aims to steer users away from illicit markets, including the likelihood of exposure to non-cannabis substances typically offered in illicit drug markets (Lenton et al., 2000; McDonald et al., 1994; Priori et al., 2002).

Belgium

In Belgium, there appears to have been a lack of legislative clarity and consequently some confusion among the general public as to what its cannabis control laws mean (see (Gelders & van der Laenen, 2007). However, prohibition with civil penalties applies, and it is reported that adults found in possession of up to 3 g of dried cannabis or resin or one plant for personal use without aggravating circumstances or signs of problematic use are eligible for a simple warning involving a police fine of 15–25 euros (Dorn, 2004; EMCDDA European Monitoring Centre for Drugs and Drug Addiction, 2007). Furthermore, it appears that the 2003 'aggravating circumstances or signs of problematic use' provisions – used as possible grounds for more punitive, that is, criminal enforcement procedures – were subsequently annulled as 'unclear' by the Belgian constitutional court and are currently not used in practice (EMCDDA European Monitoring Centre for Drugs and Drug Addiction, 2007c).

Italy

Italy was one of the first countries to depenalize cannabis (and other illicit drug) use, doing so in 1975. It has, however, changed its control policy approach several times since, repenalizing personal drug use in 1990 and depenalizing again in 1993 (Solivetti, 2001; van het Loo *et al.*, 2003). Currently, in Italy, cannabis use is regarded as an administrative offence. For cannabis use, a warning is given for the first offence on the presumption that the offender does not intend to repeat the offence in the future. For subsequent offences, an administrative penalty (such as suspension of driver's license) is given (Dorn, 2004; EMCDDA European Monitoring Centre for Drugs and Drug Addiction, 2007; Solivetti, 2001).

Czech Republic

The Czech Republic abolished offences of possession of illegal drugs for personal use in 1990. However, drug possession was again made illegal by law in 1999. In 2003, after a 2001 evaluation which showed that this policy had failed (Zabransky *et al.*, 2001, see Chapter 5), the Czech Parliament considered legislative re-classification of drugs based on an assessment of their danger to health (Zabransky, 2004). Subsequently, in March 2006, the draft law which distinguished cannabis from other psychoactive drugs in terms of its harmful consequences, and therefore provided for limited penal consequences for its use, was rejected. A renewed effort to change the penal code succeeded in the lower house of parliament in November, 2008 (Anonymous, 2008), but had not become law by March, 2009. A draft administrative decree effectively decriminalizing the possession of small amounts of cannabis and other drugs is not yet binding on the courts (Anonymous, 2008). Czech law, as it currently stands, predominantly applies administrative sanctions to cannabis possession – as well as to the possession of other illegal drugs – if the quantity in question is small (about 10 doses or 30 mg THC for cannabis products), subject to a fine or warning imposed by police. Criminal offences and jail terms of 1–5 years apply to larger possession offences (EMCDDA European Monitoring Centre for Drugs and Drug Addiction, 2007).

Portugal

Cannabis use control reforms enacted in Portugal have involved elements of both *prohibition with civil penalties* and *diversion schemes*. Portugal decriminalized – that is, removed from the ambit of criminal control – the personal possession, use and acquisition of all drugs including cannabis in 2001. The reforms, which however maintained the formal illegality of drug offences, introduced a system of referral of offenders to Commissions for the Dissuasion of Drug Addiction (CDTs), under which treatment is offered in cases where the individual is identified as having a cannabis use problem. The CDTs are established on a regional basis and comprised of a three-person panel (medical professionals, social workers, and legal advisers). Police refer offenders to the CDTs, where they must appear within 72 hours. The CDT's primary aim is to support dependent users in attending treatment, but they can also impose penalties such as fines, community service, and suspension of professional practice, and can place bans on the person attending designated places (Hughes & Stevens, 2007). In other circumstances, administrative penalties apply for personal amounts of cannabis defined as up to 10 daily doses, for example, up to 25 g of marijuana or 5 g of resin (EMCDDA European Monitoring Centre for Drugs and Drug Addiction, 2007c; Hughes & Stevens, 2007).

Denmark

As with all psychoactive drugs made illegal by law in Denmark, cannabis possession offences are punishable by a fine or imprisonment of up to 2 years at the maximum, a fine being the standard response in practice. Warnings can be issued at the discretion of the Chief Public Prosecutor's office for amounts of up to 10 g of resin or 50 g of cannabis plant material, yet a 2004 change to the law included the directive that warnings for cannabis possession offenses are only to be used in limited circumstances, and that a fine would be the norm (EMCDDA European Monitoring Centre for Drugs and Drug Addiction, 2007). Amounts for a 'police fine' range up to 135 euros for possession of an amount between 50 g and 100 g (EMCDDA European Monitoring Centre for Drugs and Drug Addiction, 2005).

Australia

'Prohibition with civil penalty' schemes operate in four Australian jurisdictions – South Australia (since 1987), the Australian Capital Territory (since 1992), the Northern Territory (since 1996), and Western Australia (since 2004) (Lenton, 2005; Lenton *et al.*, 1999a). Currently these schemes

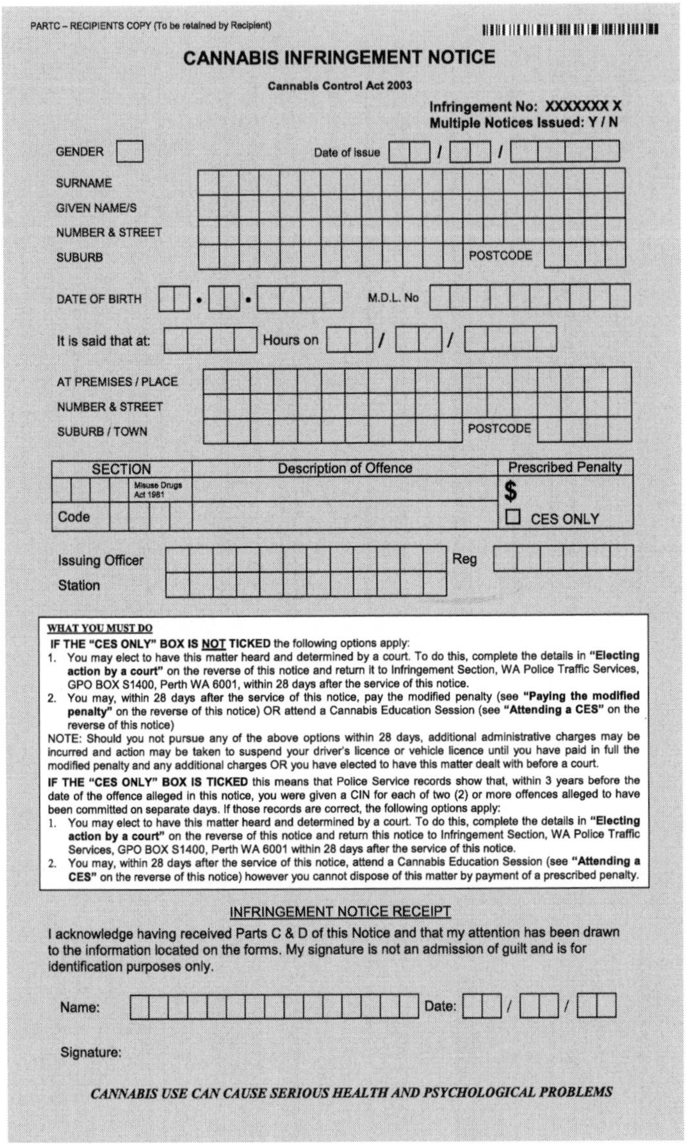

PARTC – RECIPIENTS COPY (To be retained by Recipient)

CANNABIS INFRINGEMENT NOTICE

Cannabis Control Act 2003

Infringement No: XXXXXXX X
Multiple Notices Issued: Y / N

GENDER

Date of issue / /

SURNAME

GIVEN NAME/S

NUMBER & STREET

SUBURB — POSTCODE

DATE OF BIRTH • • — M.D.L. No

It is said that at: Hours on / /

AT PREMISES / PLACE

NUMBER & STREET

SUBURB / TOWN — POSTCODE

SECTION	Description of Offence	Prescribed Penalty
Misuse Drugs Act 1981		$
Code		☐ CES ONLY

Issuing Officer — Reg

Station

WHAT YOU MUST DO

IF THE "CES ONLY" BOX IS NOT TICKED the following options apply:

1. You may elect to have this matter heard and determined by a court. To do this, complete the details in **"Electing action by a court"** on the reverse of this notice and return it to Infringement Section, WA Police Traffic Services, GPO BOX S1400, Perth WA 6001, within 28 days after the service of this notice.
2. You may, within 28 days after the service of this notice, pay the modified penalty (see **"Paying the modified penalty"** on the reverse of this notice) OR attend a Cannabis Education Session (see **"Attending a CES"** on the reverse of this notice)

NOTE: Should you not pursue any of the above options within 28 days, additional administrative charges may be incurred and action may be taken to suspend your driver's licence or vehicle licence until you have paid in full the modified penalty and any additional charges OR you have elected to have this matter dealt with before a court.

IF THE "CES ONLY" BOX IS TICKED this means that Police Service records show that, within 3 years before the date of the offence alleged in this notice, you were given a CIN for each of two (2) or more offences alleged to have been committed on separate days. If those records are correct, the following options apply:

1. You may elect to have this matter heard and determined by a court. To do this, complete the details in **"Electing action by a court"** on the reverse of this notice and return this notice to Infringement Section, WA Police Traffic Services, GPO BOX S1400, Perth WA 6001 within 28 days after the service of this notice.
2. You may, within 28 days after the service of this notice, attend a Cannabis Education Session (see **"Attending a CES"** on the reverse of this notice) however you cannot dispose of this matter by payment of a prescribed penalty.

INFRINGEMENT NOTICE RECEIPT

I acknowledge having received Parts C & D of this Notice and that my attention has been drawn to the information located on the forms. My signature is not an admission of guilt and is for identification purposes only.

Name: — Date: / /

Signature:

CANNABIS USE CAN CAUSE SERIOUS HEALTH AND PSYCHOLOGICAL PROBLEMS

Plate 4.1 Western Australian cannabis infringement notice.
Source: Reproduced from Drug and Alcohol Office (2007b).

apply to minor possession, as well as to small-scale cultivation and trafficking offences in some of these jurisdictions. There is no uniformity in the eligible amounts of cannabis for these civil penalty provisions, or in the fines imposed. Thus, at the time of writing, fines ranged from \$A50 to \$A200 per offence. The amount of harvested cannabis eligible for an infringement or expiation notice ranged from 30 g in Western Australia to 100 g in South Australia. Plant limits ranged from 2 plants (hydroponic or not) in the Northern Territory to 1 non-hydroponic plant in South Australia. However, over recent years in some jurisdictions there have been reductions in the number of plants and exclusion of hydroponic cultivated plants from the infringement notice schemes. For example, South Australia's original 10 (hydro or non-hydro) plant limit was reduced to 3 plants in 1999 (reflecting concerns about increases in yield due to increases in hydroponic cultivation), further down to 1 plant in 2000, and to 1 non-hydroponic plant in 2001 (Drug and Alcohol Office, 2007b). After the West Australian cannabis infringement notice (CIN) scheme's legislative review at the end of its first 3 years of operation, a proposal is before the WA parliament to reduce the amount of harvested cannabis eligible for an infringement notice from 30 g to 15 g, to make cultivation of 2 non-hydroponic plants no longer eligible for an infringement notice and to increase the financial penalties which apply (Drug and Alcohol Office, 2007a). Typically in these schemes there are no special provisions for repeat offenders, although in the WA scheme, those issued a notice on more than 3 occasions in a 2-year period do not have the option of paying the fine, but must attend the education session to expiate their infringement notice. In some jurisdictions (e.g. South Australia) police are required to issue an infringement notice if the person is eligible, whereas in others (e.g. Western Australia) police have the discretion to issue a notice or a criminal charge, although issuing a notice would be the norm unless the person is simultaneously charged with a serious other offence or is suspected of drug dealing (Lenton, 2005). However, a new and more conservative state government elected in 2008 has pledged to reintroduce criminal penalties for possession and growing, with a caution for first offenders applying to possession of small amounts of cannabis or a smoking implement, but not to cultivation (Spagnolo, 2009).

Partial prohibition (*de facto* or *de jure* 'legalization' of cannabis use)

General remarks

Under *Partial Prohibition* reforms, personal cannabis use and possession activities are no longer illegal, but commercial activities such as large-scale possession, production, and supply of large amounts of the drug are prohibited. Under this system, the legality of personal use amounts is usually limited to adults, and often excludes the so-called 'aggravating circumstances' which are specifically defined (e.g. use near a school or involving minors, etc.) (Macintosh, 2006; McDonald *et al.*, 1994). Importantly, *partial prohibition* regimes of cannabis possession control are brought about by two fundamentally distinct approaches, namely either (1) legalization of cannabis use by way of an expediency principle ('*de facto* legalization') or (2) *de jure* legalization of cannabis use. In the first model, cannabis use is usually prohibited by criminal law, yet formalized procedures of enforcement practice (i.e. either at the law enforcement or prosecution level) have created a situation in which personal cannabis use is predictably not sanctioned by any punitive interventions. In the second model, the legality of personal cannabis use is defined by the letter of the respective law, that is, the non-punishment of cannabis use is either explicitly written into the relevant drug control statute or the scope of the law governing illegal drug use does not extend to cannabis possession. Importantly, *de jure* legalization of cannabis use is not dependent on the way the law is applied in practice, but rather is a result of the existing legal norms.

The rationales for such reforms in the jurisdictions where they occurred all include similar elements: law and policymakers were confronted with the persistent reality of cannabis being a popular and prevalent drug across the population, the risks or harms of cannabis use were not seen as being disproportionately greater than those of alcohol or tobacco, and the approach of partial prohibition was seen as a possible way to separate cannabis use from other (more dangerous) illicit drug cultures and/or markets as well as to save criminal justice resources related to the criminal control of the drug (McDonald *et al.*, 1994; Reinarman & Cohen, 2004; MacCoun & Reuter, 1997).

De facto legalization (i.e. prohibition with an expediency principle)

The Netherlands

Cannabis possession is technically illegal and prohibited under the Dutch drug control law enshrined in the country's criminal code. Under the 'expediency principle' applying to criminal procedures, the prosecution may decide whether or not to enforce the law against certain offenses on the basis of whether this action would be 'in the public interest' (Chatwin, 2003; Duncan & Nicholson, 1997). This approach has resulted in a system of *de facto* legalization of cannabis use in the Netherlands, where personal cannabis use is actively tolerated within specific parameters, that is, not followed by sanctions or interventions. These include the home, and also the unique institution of officially sanctioned and regulated so-called *coffee shops* existing in numerous Dutch municipalities, where cannabis can openly be consumed and small amounts of cannabis (e.g. up to 5 g per day) for personal use can be purchased (Chatwin, 2003; MacCoun & Reuter, 1997; Van Dijk, 1998).

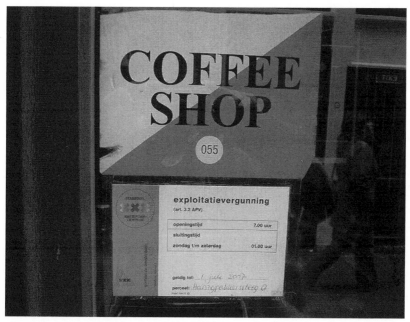

Plate 4.2 Coffee shop license displayed as required, Amsterdam.
Source: http://en.wikipedia.org/wiki/File:Coffee_shop_license_AMS_mirror.JPG

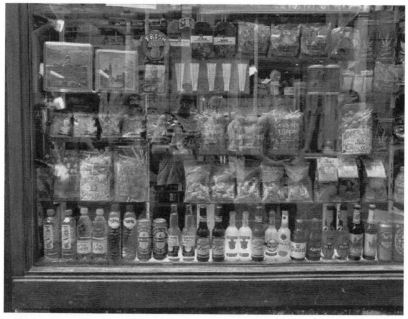

Plate 4.3 The stock-in-trade, coffee shop, Amsterdam.
Source: http://members.virtualtourist.com/m/p/m/275ebb/

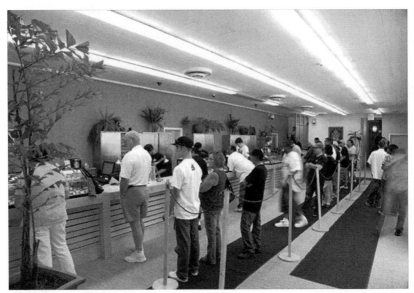

Plate 4.4 California medical cannabis dispensary (see p. 102).
Source: http://doctor2008.files.wordpress.com/2009/10/marijuana-dispensary.jpg

Cannabis use or sale outside of the regulated spaces of *coffee shops* are followed by police warnings or fines. In other words, personal cannabis use and supply to the end consumer in the Netherlands is regulated similarly to alcohol or tobacco use in many jurisdictions, and it has been suggested that this regulation scheme as applied may result in a tighter way of controlling where and how cannabis is used than punitive prohibition (Uitermark, 2004).

One of the major benefits cited for the legally tolerated provision of cannabis through the coffee shop system is that it is effecting a 'separation of drug markets', that is, that cannabis is largely traded in an environment not featuring the availability of so-called 'harder drugs', hence reducing cannabis users' possible exposure to them (MacCoun & Reuter, 1997; Pakes, 2004; Reinarman & Cohen, 2004; van Vliet, 1990). There are national guidelines about the running of the cannabis *coffee shops*, yet decisions about how they are implemented are made at the local level by a local board usually involving the mayor, the chief prosecutor, and the head of police. This 'three pillars' system means that the details of local cannabis use control policy differ from area to area, and, at least in theory, are responsive to local community concerns and interests.

While the guidelines for the retail of cannabis through the *coffee shop*, such as no sale to minors, no public nuisance, and no sale or use of other illicit drugs, have been tightened over the years and appear to work without major problems, problems have been reported with the control of the wholesale supply to the vending outlets (Polak, 1998; Uitermark, 2004). Often referred to as the 'backdoor problem' of Dutch cannabis policy, grower and supplier networks have formed to meet the existing cannabis demand, yet do not operate in a legally endorsed space or activity (de Kort & Cramer, 1999; Pakes, 2004).

This tenuous basis of the cannabis supply business is difficult for suppliers, in that they do not have access to loans or insurance or tax credits, and for regulators and enforcement, who find it hard to police a phenomenon that is necessary to respond to the tolerated personal consumption of cannabis, yet formally is illegal and violating standing law at the same time (Lenton *et al.*, 2000a). Furthermore, the Netherlands has been subjected to pressure from some of its European neighbours, the European Union, the United Nations Drug Control Program, the United States, and other countries which adopt a more prohibitionist approach to cannabis, to change its drug policy (Boekhout Van Solinge, 1999; Chatwin, 2003; 2007; Lemmens & Garretsen, 1998). The pressure has been justified on the grounds that the Netherlands policy 'undermines domestic drug policy' (e.g. in the United States), stimulates cross-border drug tourism, and undermines international collaborative efforts to reduce illicit drug use, production, and trafficking.

These pressures in recent years have also led to considerably tighter regulation of the operation of *coffee shops* and a reduction in their numbers, as well as a more stringent enforcement approach towards cannabis use outside of the tolerated areas of cannabis consumption in the Netherlands. Furthermore, commentators have observed that the current model of Dutch cannabis control policy may not be tenable or desirable in the long run, since it is based on a fundamental disjuncture between normative law and control practice, and hence the law should either be revised to reflect the given liberal practice, or be enforced in the spirit of its prohibitive norms (Uitermark, 2004).

Germany

In German law, cannabis-related offences – like all offences relating to illegal psychoactive drugs – are prohibited by the country's federal narcotics control law, and punishable by a fine or up to 5 years imprisonment. However, following the so-called 'cannabis decision' of the German Constitutional Court in 1994, subsequent to an appeal citing the disproportional approach of criminalizing cannabis use next to the legal availability of alcohol and tobacco, Germany embraced a predominant approach of *de facto* legalization of cannabis use. The main basis for this approach are chief prosecutors' directives in most of Germany's states – based on the so-called 'opportunity principle' enshrined in the German legal system – for non-prosecution of small amounts of personal cannabis possession under the drug control law. As a result of these developments in Germany, police have increasingly abstained from pro-active cannabis use enforcement, even though German law obliges them to consistently enforce the law as written, and only the prosecutor holds the formal discretion to decide against prosecution (Bollinger, 2004).

While the drug control law is a matter of federal jurisdiction, the German states ('*Länder*') are responsible for the administration of justice, and there is a considerable variation between jurisdictions in the guidelines defining how minor cannabis offences are processed under the new non-prosecution practices (Pacula *et al.*, 2005). Recent research has furthermore documented that the application of these differential guidelines has been producing rather het-erogeneous outcomes (Aulinger, 1997; Schäfer & Paoli, 2006). For example, while the maximum amount of cannabis possession eligible for non-prosecution ranges from 3 g (Baden-Württemberg) to 30 g (Schleswig-Holstein), several states' directives require non-prosecution for these amounts, whereas in the majority of states this is optional and at the discretion of the prosecutor's office on a case-by-case basis. On these grounds, it has been found that the propor-tion of cannabis possession cases which continue to be prosecuted despite being eligible for non-prosecution has ranged from 10% to 60% across states in Germany (Schäfer & Paoli, 2006). The decision as to whether prosecution should take place has been found to be most strongly influenced by the offend-er's criminal record, the number of previous offenses, substance amounts involved, and other circumstances of the offense (Schäfer & Paoli, 2006). The proportion of cannabis possession cases which are not prosecuted without any further requirements (e.g. treatment orders etc.) also varied widely, ranging from 26% to 73% across the states. The authors thus conclude that a 'consist-ent application' of current cannabis non-prosecution practices in Germany only exists in a small minority of very specific case scenarios where the offender is 'at least 20 years old, has no criminal record and the offense was not charac-terized by aggravating circumstances' (Schäfer & Paoli, 2006).

Austria

In Austria, similar to Germany, cannabis possession is, in technical terms, crimi-nally prohibited by the narcotics control law. However, on the basis of prevention and treatment clauses written into the drug law, prosecution will not take place, especially if the person has not previously come to police attention for cannabis use and is not seen to be in need of treatment. This renders personal cannabis possession largely legal on a *de facto* basis (European Database on Drugs, 2004a).

Spain

In Spain, possession or consumption of illegal psychoactive drugs – including cannabis – is technically prohibited by law, yet does not result in enforcement or punishment, especially when involving small amounts and/or use in private places (van het Loo *et al.*, 2003). Possession and use in a public place is subject to administrative sanction (e.g. suspension of driver's licence) or a fine (EMCDDA European Monitoring Centre for Drugs and Drug Addiction, 2007c). According to Gamella and Rodrigo (2004), this is the result of legal changes introduced in 1983 which decriminalized the use of all drugs and established a two-tiered legal system for production and supply of illegal drugs based on their perceived harmfulness, with cannabis in the 'softer drug' tier. However, since 1992 those carrying cannabis in public run the risk of being apprehended by police and fined. This is thought to be a key driving force behind the increasing popularity of home cultivation of cannabis since the mid-1990s (Gamella & Rodrigo, 2004).

Spanish courts have ruled that personal behaviour in a private place including private land and homes, is constitutionally protected, unless the police determine that the activities in questions are related to drug distribution (Brady, 2004). With respect to use or growing for personal use at home, there is thus effectively a situation of *de jure* legalization in Spain (see also below).

'*De jure*' legalization

United States

In 1975, the Alaska Supreme Court ruled that the state constitution's privacy protections barred the state from criminalizing adults possessing and consuming small amount of marijuana in the privacy of their homes. The legal decision thus stipulates a form of spatially restricted 'legalization' of personal use within this context. In the long legal and legislative struggle which has ensued, the courts have not strayed from this position, despite a voters' initiative to overturn it in 1991 and 2006 legislation to recriminalize possession. The issue was again back before the State Supreme Court in 2008, but the court ruled in April 2009 against making a decision on a hypothetical case (http://www.mpp.org/states/alaska/news/supreme-court-punts-pot.html).

Colombia

In *Colombia*, the personal possession of small quantities (e.g. <20 g) of any psychoactive drug is legal by law, following a Colombian Supreme Court ruling in May 1994 that the law infringed on a person's constitutional right to self-development and expression. However, as in Alaska, the political process moved to limit the effects of the decision, passing 'a series of decrees banning drug use later that same month...The decrees ban drug use almost everywhere except in the home' (Gouyis Roman *et al.*, 2005: 69).

Switzerland

In Switzerland, the currently existing federal narcotics law makes cannabis possession and use a criminal offense. The law's enforcement with regards to cannabis use differs between cantons, yet in recent years has become more restrictive, with increasing numbers of charges for personal use/possession (Eidgennössische Kommission fur Drogenfragen, 2008; van het Loo *et al.*, 2003). In 2006, more than 28,000 arrests for cannabis possession offences have been reported, constituting approximately 70% of all arrests under the narcotics law (Schweizerische Eidgenossenschaft, 2007).

A government proposal in 2001 for a comprehensive reform of the narcotics control law was to introduce *de jure* changes exempting personal cannabis possession and use from any penalties, and also to allow some cultivation and trade for personal use under certain conditions, including provision for licensed retail outlets (Schweizer Bundesrat, 2001). This proposal was introduced into the Swiss Parliament in 2003 (van het Loo *et al.*, 2003; Kapp, 2003), but rejected in 2004 (Geiser, 2007).

This proposed initiative for cannabis law reform in Switzerland may be considered unique in Western countries, in that it provided for an explicit framework that sheltered personal cannabis use from any punitive consequences by law (Fischer *et al.*, 2003). However, the initiative in the end did not find the necessary political and public support, in a situation with some indications of rising cannabis rates, for example, among Swiss teenagers, over the period of the past decade (de Preux *et al.*, 2004).

More recently, the Swiss 'Hemp Initiative' – an effort mainly driven by NGOs and diverse interest groups in the drugs field in Switzerland – was a proposal which again proposes to legalize personal cannabis use as well as to create a system of government-regulated cannabis distribution. Under the unique Swiss political system, this proposal needed to be put before a parliamentary vote and a public referendum. In March 2008, the initiative was barely defeated by both chambers of the Swiss parliament. On 30 November 2008, it was rejected by a 63% majority of voters in a referendum, while in the same vote a government proposal to institutionalize heroin maintenance was passed with a 68% majority (BBC News, 2008; Geiser, 2007; NZZ Online, 2008).

In response to the Hemp Initiative's cannabis law reform proposal, the Health Committee of the Swiss National Council (federal government) announced a counter-proposal in January 2008, which also intended to stipulate that personal cannabis possession and use for adults without risk to others would be exempt from any penalties, that is, proposing a framework of *de jure* legalization for personal cannabis use (NZZ Online, 2008). However, this proposition also did not find sufficient support within the government, and hence did not go forward. A decade-long period of drug law reform efforts in Switzerland, which has had some concrete successes, has thus had no success in the specific area of cannabis law reform.

India

In India, there are long traditions of use of cannabis in various forms for religious and medical, as well as sociable purposes. The 1961 Single Convention provided for a 25-year grace period by which time nonmedical use was to be discontinued, and accordingly the Indian Narcotic Drugs and Psychotropic Substances Act of 1985 outlawed customary use of cannabis, with the exception that drinks made from cannabis leaves (*bhang*) were allowed (Charles *et al.*, 2005). Use of such drinks is particularly associated with the celebration of the

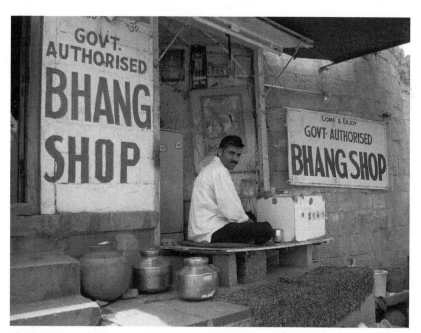

Plate 4.5 Government-licensed bhang shop, Jaisalmer, Rajasthan, India.
Source: http://en.wikipedia.org/wiki/File:Bhangshop.jpg

festival Holi in March and Baisakhi in April (Wikipedia, 2008a). Bhang is sold in a number of Indian states; travel guides list the states of Uttar Pradesh, Rajasthan, Madhya Pradesh, Uttarakhand, and Orissa (Wikitravel, 2008). The state of Rajasthan alone has 785 government-licensed bhang shops (Sharma, 2007). *Bhang lassi*, a yogurt- or milk-based drink, is the most common form, but cookies, chocolate, curries, and a smokable form can also be found on sale in shops marked as 'Government-authorized bhang shops'. As with alcohol shops in some Indian states, authorizations to run these shops are periodically sold by auction as a control measure and source of state revenue. In the Acts and Rules of the Department of Excise of the state of Uttar Pradesh, for instance, the same 'tender-cum-auction' system is specified for use for the supply of cannabis as for the supply of spirits (http://www.upexcise.in).

Spain

'Cannabis social clubs' are 'non-commercial organizations which organize the professional, collective cultivation of very limited amounts of cannabis, just enough to cover the personal needs of their club members' (Wikipedia, 2009). They have emerged in several European countries, including Belgium and Switzerland (ENCOD, 2009a). In Catalonia and the Basque country, they have achieved legal recognition and legitimation. The club in Pannagh, Bilbao has 70 members, and rents a greenhouse where the cannabis is cultivated and harvested. Every member has a right to receive a fixed amount for personal consumption, at a price set lower for medicinal than for other users, Members agree not to pass on cannabis to third persons. After a police raid and confiscation of the crop in 2005, a provincial court ruled in 2006 that there was no criminal case against the club's members or the owner of the greenhouse; the cannabis the police had confiscated was returned in 2007 to the club members (ENCOD, 2009b).

A special case: medical marijuana use control

In recent years, the regulation of so-called 'medical marijuana use' (MMU), particularly by US state provisions, has contributed to some notable legal reform arrangements of cannabis control specifically for sub-groups of individuals using cannabis for medicinal – as distinct from recreational – purposes (Hall & Degenhardt, 2003). These developments have occurred primarily in the cannabis-prohibitionist contexts of North America (e.g. Canada and several US states), more than in other Western countries. Reasons for this geographically isolated phenomenon may include that the MMU debate may not have been as salient outside of North America, as access to cannabis (purportedly) for treatment of medical conditions is more easily facilitated in the context of the cannabis reform arrangements that have occurred in many systems outside of North America (Joy *et al.*, 1999).

In essence, the main *modus operandi* of the MMU provisions in Canada and the United States is that they protect, or exempt, recognized medical marijuana users from the enforcement of standing cannabis control law that would render their cannabis use illegal and result in punishment otherwise. In other words, they establish a sub-system of 'de jure' legalization vis-à-vis MMU frameworks (an exception is the state of Maryland, where the exemption does not eliminate criminal punishment yet allows for fines, that is, relies on the use of 'administrative penalties'). Previous MMU laws which had existed in several US states were largely symbolic. The state of California enacted the first of the 'new wave' of MMU state laws in 1996 (Pacula *et al.*, 2002). The law – as most of the ones to follow in, as of December 2008, 13 states covering more than 20% of the US population – stipulated that individuals who received a recommendation from a medical doctor for marijuana use for medical purposes are allowed to grow, possess, and use limited amounts of marijuana. The law also protects specified 'caregivers' who assist in the above-mentioned activities, as well as shields doctors from federal prosecution for discussing or recommending marijuana use. The 12 other MMU states (i.e. Alaska, Colorado, Hawaii, Maine, Michigan, Montana, New Mexico, Nevada, Oregon, Rhode Island, Vermont, Washington) have created similar laws in the following years, most of which define a list of specified illnesses for which medical marijuana use might be recommended and hence result in protection from enforcement. Some of the states by now also operate formal registry programmes of sanctioned medical marijuana users (Marijuana Policy Project, 2007).

In Canada, the so-called 'Medical Marijuana Access Program' (MMAP) was established by the federal government in 2001 in the wake of a ruling by the Ontario Superior Court concluding that the blanket prohibition of cannabis use violated constitutional rights for individuals deriving medical benefits from marijuana use (Lucas, 2008; Manfredi & Maioni, 2002). Through the MMAP, medical marijuana users need to apply – on the basis of medical documentation – for exemption from criminal prosecution for both personal use and production of limited quantities of marijuana. In 2003, the Canadian MMAP was – again through the ruling of a higher court – forced to establish a government-sponsored supply of marijuana for individuals approved for medical use who were unable to find other ways of legally obtaining the drug (Lucas, 2008). Since its inception, only several hundred individuals have been approved under the MMAP. The programme has been criticized for its lengthy application process and restrictive criteria, as well as for approved users' inability to obtain customized marijuana strains from governmental sources. These problems have allegedly led many medical marijuana users in Canada to continue their MMU without a formal exemption provided by the MMAP (Health Canada, 2005; Sibbald, 2002).

The evidence in a recent investigative report on medical marijuana in California (Samuels, 2008) suggests that the scheme has grown into something close to *de facto* legalization (see Plate 4.4 on p. 94). There are more than 200,000 Californians with a medical letter from a doctor entitling them to purchase cannabis, and hundreds of dispensaries selling it. An owner of one of these estimated that 40% of her clients suffer from serious illnesses such as cancer, AIDS, glaucoma, epilepsy, and multiple sclerosis. The rest have ailments like anxiety, sleeplessness, attention deficit disorder, and assorted pains (Samuels, 2008). Despite a continuing 'low-level civil war with the federal government' in the form of the Drug Enforcement Administration, a stable grey market has emerged, with entrepreneurs avoiding trouble by following such rules as: don't advertise, don't sell to minors or cops, and don't open more than two stores. Though cannabis sold through the dispensaries is only a small fraction of the total California cannabis market, it is reported that the wholesale price of good cannabis has fallen by half since the legalization of medical marijuana (Samuels, 2008).

Reform beyond permitting cannabis use: regulating availability

In cannabis control reform regimes where cannabis use is depenalized or even permitted on a *de facto* or *de jure* basis, as in the reform systems in the countries outlined above, the supply and availability of cannabis for the purpose of personal possession and use inevitably becomes a key practical matter. This is an especially challenging issue, since most standing drug control laws in these reform systems strictly prohibit and provide for heavy punishment for any cannabis supply activities (and in some instances have been strengthened further in exchange for more liberal control approaches to dealing with possession or use), and thus by default may expose most users to considerable criminal enforcement and consequences which the alternative use control measures are aiming to reduce or avoid. Conversely, some cannabis reform regimes have included reduced penalties, such as a limited civil-law fine, for cultivation of a small number of plants for personal use – as in the existing Australian civil penalty schemes, or in the proposed Canadian cannabis use reform law (Swensen, 2007a; Fischer *et al.*, 2003).

Yet there have been several other proposals which have taken the issue further and recommended for controlled or regulated cannabis availability schemes to be put into place as a complementary measure to legal control reform regimes aiming at use/possession. Under a regulated cannabis availability system all cultivation, sale, and supply of cannabis would be controlled or regulated by the government to a greater or lesser extent, for example, either by the government carrying out an active monopoly for cannabis production and distribution (e.g. via state-owned production facilities and/or outlets), or by way of regulating and licensing designated private or commercial producers and distribution outlets. Any cultivation or distribution occurring outside the government regulated system would likely be illegal and subject to criminal sanction (McDonald *et al.*, 1994). Such a licensing or monopoly system would resemble the systems by which alcohol production and dissemination is handled in a large number of jurisdictions (Babor *et al.*, 2003).

Considerations in a system of regulated availability

That which is prohibited cannot easily be regulated. Examples can be found of efforts by the state to regulate even a prohibited market. A number of governments require sex workers to pay taxes on their earnings, even if the behaviour is defined as illegal (West, 2000). In the latter stages of state alcohol prohibition in Mississippi, spirits sales were taxed even if they were illegal (Holder & Cherpitel, 1996). And, of course, the Dutch 'coffee shops' are highly regulated in a circumstance in which what they are doing is formally illegal but officially tolerated. Despite these examples, there is no doubt that making a market legal greatly increases the mechanisms available to the state for regulating it. And those who hold a license or other permission from the state to operate in the legal market have a shared interest in putting the illegal actors out of business.

Worldwide, at the present time there are few working examples of cannabis supply regulation, though several have been proposed (see Haden, 2004). Under the Dutch system of '*de facto* legalization', the retail dissemination of cannabis in 'coffee shops' is regulated by state authorities, but not the production (Lenton *et al.*, 2000a; MacCoun & Reuter, 1997; Pakes, 2004). A recent Senate inquiry in Canada recommended that a system of government controlled cultivation and distribution of cannabis for recreational purposes be implemented in conjunction with the legalization of personal cannabis use (Senate Special Committee on Illegal Drugs, 2002). The government-sponsored reforms specific to cannabis use proposed as part of the narcotics control law revisions in Switzerland in 2004 included provisions for state-regulated cannabis availability and dissemination in conjunction with the proposed *de jure* legalization of personal cannabis use (Fischer *et al.*, 2003). The state-authorized bhang shops in Indian states are functioning examples of such systems, and studies of them would be of international interest. The state-sanctioned existing distribution systems for medical cannabis users (e.g. cannabis buyers' clubs) in Canada and the United States are another operating model of regulated cannabis availability, albeit limited to the special sub-population of medical cannabis users (Hall & Degenhardt, 2003; Lucas, 2008). These private facilities are granted permission from the state to distribute cannabis products to individuals recognized as medical cannabis users. The Canadian MMAP features an additional detail of interest, in that the federal government itself operates a cannabis cultivation facility (in an abandoned underground mine in Flin-Flan, Manitoba), which produces cannabis offered for distribution to participants in the MMAP.

Any framework of cannabis control will have its advantages and disadvantages. The experience with alcohol and tobacco regulation provides some guidance or models of what to do and what not to do. Lax regulations on sellers, self-regulation, and promotion by industry-driven commercial interests would be highly likely to produce undesirable outcomes in terms of levels of cannabis use and harm. If the risks of regulating cannabis in a legal market are to be reduced, there are several potential challenges which have to be addressed.

Changing laws to allow regulated availability of cannabis would be a relatively inexpensive process, but providing the regulatory and enforcement mechanisms to reap the benefits of an effectively regulated system will be far more expensive. Examples from other areas of drug regulation such as restriction of tobacco sales to minors and liquor licence enforcement (e.g. Loxley *et al.*, 2005) suggest that despite the promises, regulation, and enforcement is often underfunded and less effective as a result. In a legal market, cannabis is likely to be taxed, in part as a mild discouragement of use. It is highly desirable that some of this revenue be earmarked for enforcement of the regulations of the cannabis market.

Particularly at first, regulation is unlikely to completely eliminate the illicit cannabis market. The extent to which the illicit market for cannabis is undermined will likely depend on the type of regulatory system employed (McDonald *et al.*, 1994: 64). An illicit market is likely to survive if the price of cannabis is kept high or there are strict restrictions on users being able to access legal cannabis. Thus schemes for legalizing alcohol at the end of US Prohibition were careful to ensure that the legal market offered effective competition with the illicit market (Fosdick & Scott, 1933). As Haden notes, 'a drug whose production is simple and widely available indicates the need for less restrictive regulatory mechanisms in order to challenge the economic realities of the black market' (Haden, 2004: 228).

As the illicit market in cannabis will continue to exist to some degree in parallel to regulated cannabis availability, the need for criminal justice enforcement will remain, although there will be a substantial reduction in criminal justice costs from a regulated system.

Those responsible for the design, implementation, and evaluation of a potential legal, regulated model for cannabis will need to address factors such as these which may undermine the effectiveness and public and political acceptability of any such scheme.

Conclusions

1 Cannabis use control reforms which have been implemented in different countries are not always easy to get detail on or to categorize cleanly according to the reform typologies proposed in our examination. Even within clearly defined parameters of legal cannabis control, legal provisions and their implementation change over time, vary within jurisdictions, and can also hinge considerably on discretionary practices used by relevant authorities (e.g. institutions of the criminal justice system).

2 The main thrust of cannabis use control reforms observed has been towards less severe penalties for personal cannabis use, which can be expressed in either the quality (e.g. whether criminal or non-criminal) or the quantity (e.g. amount of fine) of penalties imposed. In many instances, however, traditional forms of punishment have been replaced by other behavioural requirements of the user, for example, diversion to education or treatment. Few systems do not impose any penalties at all on cannabis users.

3 A key conceptual distinction for cannabis control reform systems is whether alternative regimes are brought about by the so-called *de facto* or *de jure* mechanics. In the former, reforms are brought about by changes in how existing – usually conventional criminal – cannabis control law is applied. Such reforms then do not necessarily reflect the spirit or letter of the existing law, relying rather on discretion, and may be considered temporary or not solidly founded in the material base of law. The latter reform approaches are enshrined in law, and as such are an outcome of legislative or constitutional processes. As such, they represent a more explicit expression of existing norms regarding cannabis use, as well as offering greater predictability of consequences for cannabis users.

4 While quite a number of countries have implemented reform measures aiming at cannabis use control, fewer have addressed the issue of supply, often for political reasons. These issues are inevitably linked, since the use of cannabis requires that the product is obtained either by one's own

cultivation, by trade or by purchase. In traditional criminal control systems, but also in many reform systems, these activities are subject to heavy penalties and hence potentially expose the cannabis user to these consequences for supply activities, while the penalties for consumption are reduced. The link between use and supply thus remains a major policy challenge.

An Afterword, September 2009

In the course of 2009, there has been a substantial "breakthrough" (Jenkins, 2009) concerning various forms of decriminalization in Latin America. In February, a Latin American Commission on Drugs and Democracy, cochaired by former presidents of Brazil, Mexico and Colombia, called for a "paradigm shift" in drug policies, including examination of the decriminalization of possession of cannabis for personal use (Cardoso, 2009). Mexican legislation enacted on 20 August provides that those found carrying relatively small quantities of cannabis, cocaine, heroin or other drugs for "personal and immediate use" will be referred to free treatment programs rather than criminalized. Those caught with drugs for the third time would be forced to go to treatment, though no penalties are specified for noncompliance (Lacey, 2009). Less than a week later, in a case involving five young men arrested with a few cannabis cigarettes in their pockets, the Supreme Court of Argentina ruled that it was unconstitutional to punish people for possessing cannabis for personal consumption (BBC, 2009). The Argentinian Congress is expected to introduce amendments to current laws in support of the court decision. Brazil and Ecuador are also expected to take new decriminalizing steps (Jenkins, 2009).

Chapter 5

The impacts of cannabis policy reforms within the current drug control regime

Introduction

Background

This chapter reviews the existing evidence on the impact on cannabis use and other indicators of the alternative regimes of cannabis control which have been implemented within the current constraints of the international drug conventions. As noted in the preceding chapter, in a number of countries, at both a national and subnational level, governments have introduced changes to the policies and laws applying to cannabis.

The reforms that are generally agreed to have been conducted within the bounds of the existing international drug treaties and conventions (e.g. Krajewski, 1999), can be broadly seen as moving away from *prohibition with strict criminal penalties* on the user (full prohibition) to some form of depenalization. As described in detail in the previous chapter, the reform typologies include: *prohibition with cautioning or diversion*; *prohibition with civil penalties* (often termed 'decriminalization'); *partial prohibition*, including both '*de facto*' and '*de jure*' legalization; and *regulated availability of cannabis as a medicine*, often referred to as 'medical marijuana'. While not all of these reforms have been extensively evaluated, there is a small but growing evidence base, and this is the focus of the present chapter.

Caveats and data limitations

Caution needs to be exercised in interpreting the published evidence evaluating the impact of cannabis policies for a number of reasons.

First, the policy environment is a dynamic one where effects decay and the policy that is implemented changes over time (see Pacula *et al.*, 2005). This is important from the point of view of single longitudinal studies, as results may be affected by formal legislative and procedural changes as well as informal law enforcement practices (see Kilmer, 2002). When trying to make sense of the results of comparative reviews, one needs to clarify the cannabis law and its implementation in a location at the time that the review was conducted.

Secondly, international comparisons are difficult and results can be confounded by cultural, political, geographic, and climatic differences.

Thirdly, cannabis law reform often occurs in locations with high rates of use. This means that pre-post or longitudinal designs with 'matched' control locations are needed to identify true impacts on rates of cannabis use. Simply creating a dummy 'decriminalized' variable and comparing rates of use in so-called 'decriminalized' versus 'non-decriminalized' states, without adjusting for pre-change rates of cannabis use, will run the risk of erroneously concluding that 'decriminalized' states have higher rates of cannabis use *because* of the policy change. Causation may in fact go in the other direction: policy may have been liberalized precisely because of high rates of use and experiences of people being prosecuted under the law.

Fourthly, evaluations rarely take into account the level of knowledge in the community about the laws which apply to cannabis (Pacula *et al.*, 2005). Levels of knowledge may vary in the general community, in occasional and in regular cannabis users in ways that may influence how changes to the law affect rates of cannabis use.

Finally, any research evidence may not predict the effects of new reforms in other locations, because the impacts of future cannabis policy reforms may depend on contextual factors and on how the reforms are implemented. Therefore it remains important that any changes to cannabis policy are evaluated, and their effects monitored and used to review their performance.

To date, research has focused on three outcome domains:

(i) *General deterrence effects* – the impact of changing the law on rates of cannabis use in (a) the general community; and (b) among the young – who are seen as the most vulnerable to any adverse health (and particularly mental health) effects of regular cannabis use (Arseneault *et al.*, 2002; Coffey *et al.*, 2002; Lubman *et al.*, 2007; Smit *et al.*, 2004; Winters & Lee, 2008).

(ii) *Specific deterrence effects* – the impacts on the cannabis use of those who have been apprehended.

(iii) *Adverse social impacts* of the system of control on apprehended users. Few studies have looked at: impacts on harms, the drug market or sentinel groups such as regular users, who may be more likely to show adverse effects that are less evident in general population studies.

In this short review we have refrained from going to original sources of data such as prevalence statistics and attempting to draw conclusions about what they can tell us about the impact of cannabis reforms or otherwise. Given the heterogeneous patterns of reform, the difficulties in identifying implementation practices, and the existence and impact of extraneous non-legal factors, we have limited ourselves to considering those examples of cannabis law reforms where detailed studies have been conducted by authors with knowledge and insights into the range of country- and region-specific issues which need to be taken into account when trying to understand the impact of such reforms.

Evidence on impacts of reforms

Most of the published research has evaluated the impact of moving from *strict prohibition* to *prohibition with civil penalties*. This has primarily been by comparing outcomes of policy changes in different states in the United States and Australia. A few studies have evaluated the impact of the Netherlands' *prohibition with an expediency principle scheme*. There are at least four studies on the *economic impacts* of such changes and one or two on the wider impacts of *medical marijuana initiatives* in North America.

Policy impact studies

United States

Impacts on rates of use

At least four uncontrolled studies and four studies employing matched control states were conducted to measure the impact on rates of use of the changes in state cannabis law that occurred in the United States from 1973 to 1978. Although data from the uncontrolled studies were used to support the changes, interpretation of the results of these studies was problematic and for that reason we focus here on the controlled studies. Taken together, these four studies indicated that states which introduced reforms did not experience greater increases in cannabis use among adults or adolescents. Nor did surveys in these states show more favourable attitudes towards cannabis use than those states which maintained strict prohibition with criminal penalties (Single, 1989; Single *et al.*, 2000; Theis & Register, 1993).

In a study not designed to measure the impact of cannabis 'decriminalization', Stuart and colleagues (Stuart *et al.*, 1976) conducted a policy impact study of change in cannabis use sanctions in Ann Arbor, Michigan. They found that cannabis use was not affected by several changes in the municipal cannabis laws, including imposing a maximum penalty of $5 fine for cannabis use, compared to three neighbouring communities in Michigan which did not reduce penalties for use of the drug.

Saveland and Bray (1981) conducted secondary analyses of four national drug use surveys between 1972 and 1977. They found that cannabis use was higher in the 'decriminalized' states, both before *and* after the changes in law. Those that did moderate their law had increasing rates of use among adolescents and adults, but this was greater in the 'non-decriminalization' states, and the greatest proportional increase in use was in the states with the most severe penalties. However, the 'decriminalized' states employed by the authors were California, Maine, Minnesota, Ohio, and Rhode Island. The last of these was not strictly one of the 11 'decriminalized' states because, while it reduced the penalties for cannabis use, it still allowed the possibility of imprisonment (Single, 1989). However, its small population size meant that it was unlikely to affect the results.

The third controlled study used data from Monitoring the Future national surveys of high-school students. Oversampling high-school students in the decriminalized states and comparing trends in them with trends elsewhere, Johnson and colleagues (e.g. Johnston *et al.*, 1981) concluded that decriminalization had no effect on either the rates of cannabis use, or related attitudes and beliefs about cannabis use, among this age group.

In a more recent study of the effects of the legal status imposed by individual states for possession of a small amount of cannabis, Theis and Register (1993) conducted a logistic regression analysis of a sample of 3,913 males in the National Longitudinal Survey of Youth who were between the ages of 14 and 21 in 1979 and were reinterviewed in 1984 and 1988. Controlling for a range of factors including age, education, marital status, ethnicity, urbanisation, parents' education, and religious participation, income and wealth, and 'well-being', they found 'no strong evidence' that cannabis 'decriminalization' affected the choice, frequency, or use of alcohol, cannabis, or cocaine.

These controlled studies are very dated but, for reasons already noted, there are problems with conducting analyses of more contemporary data to determine the 'impact' on current cannabis use of changes to cannabis laws which occurred decades earlier in these states. Pacula and colleagues (Pacula *et al.*, 2003; 2005) concluded, after reviewing state laws from 1989 to 1999, that some (Alaska, California, North Carolina, and Arizona) of the so-called decriminalized states could no longer be classed as 'decriminalized', and a number of previously 'non-decriminalized' states had effectively removed criminal penalties (Louisiana, Massachusetts, New Jersey, Vermont, Wisconsin, and West Virginia). According to Pacula *et al.*, there were 15 'decriminalized' states in 1999, and a further 13 of the so-called 'non-decriminalized' states had introduced cautioning and diversion schemes. Thus, analyses of rates of cannabis use a decade or more after the changes in the original 11 'decriminalization' states will be confounded by these effects.

Impacts on other indicators of harm

A small number of studies have tried to measure impacts of the 'decriminalization' of cannabis on indicators of harm. For example, Model (1993), who
conducted a study of hospital emergency room data from 1975 to 1978, suggested that 'decriminalization' of cannabis in the 12 states was accompanied by
a significant decrease in emergency room episodes involving drugs other than
cannabis, and an increase in cannabis episodes. Her interpretation was that
when cannabis was depenalized, illicit drug users tended to stay with the use of
cannabis, and move away from the use of the other more severely punished
illicit drugs.

Australia

Evaluations have been conducted on the *prohibition with cautioning* and *prohibition with civil penalties* schemes that have been in place in the eight Australian
states and territories. However, evaluations of the cautioning and diversion
schemes have been exclusively process evaluations (e.g. Hales *et al.*, 2004).
They have not looked at the impact of these changes on rates of cannabis use,
and for that reason are not considered further here. A number of studies of
impacts on rates of use have been conducted comparing Australian jurisdictions which have introduced civil penalties for minor cannabis offences and
those which have not. The South Australian Cannabis Expiation Notice (CEN)
system, which commenced in 1987, is the longest running and most researched
Australian scheme.

Impacts on rates of use

An analysis of national population survey data conducted as part of an evaluation of the South Australian Scheme indicated that over the 10-year period
from 1985 there had been an increase in self-reported lifetime cannabis use
among persons aged 14 years and over, in all states and territories, with a
greater degree of increase in South Australia than in the average of the other
Australian jurisdictions (Donnelly *et al.*, 1999; 2000). Between 1985 and 1995,
the adjusted prevalence rates of ever having used cannabis increased in South
Australia from 26% to 36%. There were also significant increases in Victoria
(from 26% to 32%), Tasmania (from 21% to 33%), and New South Wales
(from 26% to 33%), all of which had maintained strict prohibition of cannabis
use. However, jurisdictions also differed in rates of change, with Victoria and
Tasmania having similar rates of increase to South Australia (Donnelly *et al.*,
1999; 2000). The analysis failed to find a statistically significant difference
between South Australia and the rest of Australia in the rate of increase in
weekly cannabis use. This suggested that even if South Australians were slightly

more likely to have ever tried cannabis than Australians in other jurisdictions, this did not result in higher rates of regular use in that state (Donnelly *et al.*, 1999; 2000).

Although the introduction of the CEN scheme in South Australia did not apply to juveniles, there was some apprehension that a liberalization of the laws might encourage cannabis use by young people. To examine this possibility, two groups examined data from three thousand South Australian students aged 11 to 16 years surveyed in 1986, 1987, 1988, and 1989 (Donnelly *et al.*, 1992; Neill *et al.*, 1991). Cannabis consumption levels in this age group remained stable between 1986 and 1989, with 20% saying that they had ever tried cannabis and 6% having used within the last week (Neill *et al.*, 1991). On the basis of this analysis, it did not appear that changes to the cannabis laws impacted on cannabis use by secondary school students. Unfortunately, there were no data available concerning the prevalence of cannabis use among teenagers not attending school, who may have been more likely to engage in cannabis use compared to those remaining in formal education.

Donnelly *et al.* (1999; 2000) also analysed trends in cannabis use among 14 to 29 year olds, the age group with the highest rates of initiation and regular cannabis use (Donnelly & Hall, 1994). Their analysis concluded that there had been an Australia-wide increase in rates of lifetime cannabis use between 1985 and 1995 in this age group, but that the rate of increase in lifetime cannabis use in South Australia did not differ from that in the rest of Australia. Indeed, the South Australia rate was in the middle of the range of rates found among the different jurisdictions in the 1995 survey (Donnelly *et al.*, 1999; 2000). Regarding recent use, these authors also failed to find any consistent trends in rates of weekly cannabis use among 14 to 29 year olds in any jurisdictions from 1988 to 1995. However, they concluded that much larger samples would be needed definitively to rule out the possibility that there had been small differences in rates of increase among young people between jurisdictions (Donnelly *et al.*, 1999).

Overall, Donnelly and colleagues concluded that the increase in lifetime cannabis use in South Australia was unlikely to be due to the implementation of the Cannabis Expiation Notice Scheme, because: (1) similar increases occurred in Tasmania and Victoria, where the legal status of cannabis use did not change during the same period; (2) weekly cannabis use in South Australia did not increase at faster rate than the rest of Australia; and (3) there was no greater increase in cannabis use among young adults aged 14 to 29 years, which is the age group with the highest rates of initiation of cannabis use, in South Australia (Donnelly *et al.*, 1999; 2000).

In a study of the impact of the Simple Cannabis Offence Notice (SCON) scheme which came into effect in the Australian Capital Territory (ACT) in

1992, McGeorge and Aitken (1997) compared pre (1992) and post (1994) rates of cannabis use among 221 university students in the ACT with a control group of 246 university students in Victoria, which had maintained a strict criminal penalty scheme. Prevalence of lifetime cannabis use remained stable at about 53% over time, and frequency of use was indistinguishable between the two sites. The authors concluded that decriminalization of cannabis had no effect on rates of cannabis use.

Surveys investigating the impact of the Western Australian CIN scheme (which came into effect in March 2004, and is the most recent of the Australian civil penalty schemes) suggested that cannabis use in that state has not increased since the scheme's inception. Use in the past year among those aged 14 to 70 decreased from 18% in 2002 to 12% in 2007. The authors do not claim that these reductions were due to the CIN scheme itself, because similar declines have occurred in other Australian jurisdictions and this trend began a number of years before the CIN scheme came into effect (Fetherston & Lenton, 2007).

Williams and colleagues (Cameron & Williams, 2001; Williams, 2004; Williams & Mahmoudi, 2004) conducted a small number of omnibus studies on the impact of the Australian civil penalty schemes. They used data from the five national drug household surveys conducted in Australia from 1988 to 1998, along with police seizure data and other sources, to determine the impact of criminal and non-criminal sanctions on decisions to use cannabis. For example, Williams (2004) concluded, after controlling for cannabis price, level of police enforcement, propensities to use and other factors, that the decision to use cannabis by males over the age of 25 was affected by changes in legal penalties in South Australia, the Australian Capital Territory, and the Northern Territory. But there was no evidence that 'decriminalization' significantly increased initiation to cannabis use by young males or females, or the frequency of use among existing users. However, a problem with these studies is that, in comparing cannabis prevalence and frequency rates in 'decriminalized' vs 'non-decriminalized states', they failed to take into account that rates of cannabis use are typically higher in jurisdictions which introduce civil penalties well *before* the reforms are put in place. Thus, the limited finding that prevalence of 'ever' using cannabis was higher in those states that had introduced civil penalty schemes does not mean that this was due to the legal reforms. It is also open to the alternative interpretation: that older adults are less likely to deny earlier use of cannabis if criminal penalties for use have been removed.

Social impacts of civil versus criminal penalties

Lenton and colleagues (Lenton *et al.*, 1999; 2000) compared the social impacts of a conviction under strict cannabis prohibition in place at the time in Western

Australia with that of an infringement notice under the CEN system in South Australia. They did so by comparing the experiences of 68 matched first-time apprehended cannabis users from each of these states. Although based on self-selected convenience samples rather than randomly selected cannabis offenders, this study remains one of few to have documented the social impacts of conviction versus civil penalty for a minor cannabis offence. Those in the WA convicted group were significantly more likely than the South Australian infringement notice group to report: adverse employment consequences (32% vs 2%); further contact with the criminal justice system (32% vs 0%); relationship problems (20% vs 5%), and accommodation difficulties (16% vs 0%) that could be attributed to their apprehension for the cannabis offence (Lenton et al., 1999; 2000). The study failed to find a significant difference between the groups in terms of negative travel effects of conviction or infringement notice (0% vs 7%). This was possibly because the time from apprehension to interview (average 38 months) may not have been long enough for any effects on travel to be evident in a large enough number of the convicted sample to result in a significant finding (Lenton et al., 1999; 2000).

Lenton and colleagues (Lenton et al., 1999; 2000) also found that neither the infringement notice nor the cannabis conviction appeared to have much impact on subsequent cannabis use. Around 91% of the South Australian infringement notice group and 71% of the Western Australian convicted group said that their cannabis use one month afterwards was 'not at all' affected by their apprehension. Rates of post-apprehension cannabis use were highly correlated with rates of use prior to apprehension, consistent with other research (e.g. Erickson, 1976; 1980).

Cannabis users arrested and convicted for the first time in Western Australia were more likely to report negative attitudes to police and the justice system than their South Australian counterparts who received an infringement notice. Thus, 49% of the Western Australian group, compared with only 18% of the expiators, said that they had become less trusting of police, and 43% of the Western Australian convicted group, compared to 15% of the South Australian expiators, were more fearful of police as a result. The greater loss of trust in the Western Australian sample appeared in part due to the greater number of that group who were apprehended in a private residence, but did not appear to be due to other possible confounders (Lenton et al., 1999; 2000).

Research has also been conducted in Australia on the impact of introducing prohibition with civil penalty schemes on public attitudes and knowledge. Three main conclusions can be drawn.

1 In Australian states which have prohibition with civil penalty schemes, even after these schemes have been in place for a number of years, the

majority of the public support the use of non-criminal penalties for minor cannabis users, even if there may be a small reduction of support for the measures from pre-change levels. For example, in South Australia a public attitude sample conducted 10 years after the introduction of the CEN scheme found that 57% thought the laws should remain as they are or become less strict, compared to 38% who thought they should be more strict (Heale *et al.*, 2000). In Western Australia the proportion of the public who thought the Cannabis Infringement Notice Scheme introduced in 2004 was 'a good idea' fell significantly from 79% in 2002 to 66% in 2007, but, despite this drop, two-thirds still supported the scheme (Fetherston & Lenton, 2007).

2 In Australian states where such schemes have been introduced, a larger proportion of the population than in states where criminal penalties apply mistakenly believe that cannabis use has been legalized (Fitzsimmons & Cooper-Stanbury, 2000).

3 There is no evidence that cannabis is seen as *less* harmful in those states once civil penalties were introduced. Indeed, in Western Australia, Fetherston and Lenton (2007) found that the WA public saw cannabis use as more harmful to health in 2007 than they did in 2002 before the scheme was introduced. Again, this was not to say that the more negative views towards cannabis occurred *because* of the legal changes, as attitudes to cannabis had been becoming progressively more negative since well before the legal changes among both adults (Draper & Serafino, 2006) and school children (Miller & Lang, 2007). Rather, there was no evidence of cannabis being seen as more benign.

Problems with civil penalty schemes

There were three major problems associated with the cannabis infringement notice system that was implemented in South Australia. First, only 45% of people paid their fines by the due date (Christie & Ali, 2000). Secondly, there was 2.5-fold increase in the number of people who were issued notices from 1987–1988 to 1993–1994. This so-called 'net-widening' appeared to be largely due to the ease with which notices could be issued by police. Its effect was to increase the numbers at risk of criminal sanction for non-payment of fines, an outcome that can particularly disadvantage those with limited financial means (Christie & Ali, 2000). Thirdly, there was evidence that criminal gangs were syndicating cannabis cultivation by aggregating for sale multiple crops of cannabis plants that individuals were growing under the original 10-plant limit (Sutton & McMillan, 2000).

Recent evaluation of the first three years of the CIN scheme in Western Australia suggests that features of this scheme may have addressed these problems. While only 43% of people expiate their notice by the due date, a further 25% were expiated in the 1–2 months afterwards, because non-payers risked the sanction of losing their driver's licence if the notice wasn't expiated. The overall expiation rate, allowing for delayed payment beyond the 1–2 month period, is estimated at up to 75% (Drug and Alcohol Office, 2007a). It appears that the additional time to pay and further penalty provided through this administrative sanction may contribute to the higher overall expiation rate. While there has been some net-widening in the scheme, this only resulted in an overall increase in total consequences by some 14% (compared to 250% in the SA case), 90% of which was due to the inclusion of implement offences (possession of bongs, etc.) within the CIN scheme (Drug and Alcohol Office, 2007b). Furthermore, under the WA scheme, only two plants per primary residence are eligible for an infringement notice. This, in addition to other aspects of the scheme (such as providing support for police to charge people they believe are using the infringement levels as a cover for dealing activities, and reducing the cut-off for being deemed a supplier from 25 to 10 plants) seems to have prevented the exploitation of the plant limit by syndicating growing that was seen under the SA scheme (see Sutton & McMillan, 2000).

Another problem with civil penalty schemes is that they can cause disproportionate hardship for already socially and economically disadvantaged members of society. Early work on the South Australian scheme indicated that socially disadvantaged persons were over-represented among those failing to pay expiation fines (Sarre *et al.*, 1989). Studies conducted since that time show that attempts to reduce the financial burden of fines have had some success (Christie & Ali, 2000; Drug and Alcohol Office, 2007b). However, data from the first three years of operation of the Western Australian scheme show that indigenous people continue to be disadvantaged by new penalty options, and are six times less likely to expiate their notice than their non-indigenous counterparts. Special effort needs to be made to monitor and address this problem by those implementing civil penalty schemes (Lenton, 2007).

Portugal

Hughes and Stevens (2007) reviewed available literature and statistics and conducted stakeholder interviews to understand the impacts of the Portuguese reforms introduced in 2001. As described in the previous chapter, these reforms removed criminal sanctions for personal possession, use and acquisition of all drugs including cannabis, and introduced a system of diversion to Commissions for the Dissuasion of Drug Addiction (CDTs). Hughes and Stevens (2007) concluded that: (i) changes in reported patterns of cannabis, and other drug use patterns were apparent, but it was unclear whether these changes were real and, if so, whether they were due to the policy reforms or to more reflective of Europe-wide trends in drug use, such as those that occurred in Spain and Italy, which did not change the law; (ii) there had been increases in numbers of people attending for cannabis treatment; (iii) there had been difficulties with the operation of the Community Drug Treatment centres (CDTs); and (iv) there were views at a political level about changes needed to the reforms which ranged from scrapping them to streamlining the operation of the CDTs and increasing resources for treatment services.

General population surveys of the Portuguese public only commenced in 2001, the same year the reforms were introduced, and there are no recent data series at the population level to monitor changes since that time. However, surveys of school students have been conducted as part of the European School Survey Project on Alcohol and Other Drugs (ESPAD), with surveys in 1999 and 2003. These data indicate an increase in self-reported cannabis use among 16–18 year olds in Portugal from 9.4% in 1999 to 15.1% in 2003. However, Hughes and Stevens note that school surveys such as these are often susceptible to reporting bias, and they thought that decriminalization may have led young people to be more willing to admit to cannabis use in such surveys (Hughes & Stevens, 2007).

Official treatment statistics show a reduction in heroin-related treatment presentations and an increase in cannabis presentations. Thus, referrals to the CDTs for cannabis increased from 47% in 2001 to 67% in 2003, and stayed at around that level in the two years thereafter. Heroin presentations, by contrast, dropped from 33% in 2001 to 17% in 2003 and have remained fairly stable since. Importantly, while the CDTs have been seen as crucial to the success of the reform process, they have also been criticized as being too administratively cumbersome and resource intensive. The Portuguese reforms have highlighted the need for a well-operating referral and treatment system (Hughes & Stevens, 2007).

In conclusion, these authors state:

> The Portuguese experience cannot provide a definitive guide to the effects of decriminalization of drugs, but only indications of the results of decriminalization in the specific Portuguese context. It is not possible to tell the extent to which changes were caused by decriminalization or the wider drug strategy. The extent to which difficulties in implementation impeded the impacts from the reform remains unclear.
>
> (Hughes & Stevens, 2007: 9)

United Kingdom

The UK government reclassified cannabis as a Class C drug on 29 January 2004. In July 2007 the question of reclassifying cannabis as a Class B drug was referred to the Advisory Council on the Misuse of Drugs (ACMD). Despite the fact that the ACMD, having reviewed the available evidence, believed that cannabis should remain a Class C drug (Advisory Council on the Misuse of Drugs, 2008), the British Government rejected this advice and, consistent with a number of statements by Prime Minister Gordon Brown, decided to reclassify cannabis as a Class B drug (Castle, 2008).

We found no evidence of the 2004 reclassification leading to an increase in cannabis use. Indeed, data from the British Crime Survey suggests that while the number of police contacts for cannabis use increased, cannabis use decreased. Police contacts for possession of cannabis increased from 88,263 in 2004–2005 to 119,917 in 2005–2006 and 130,406 in 2006–2007 (Nicholas *et al.*, 2007: 40), which the authors noted may reflect changes such as 'the use of formal warnings for cannabis, rather than real changes in its incidence' (p. 21), particularly as these street warnings counted towards Home Office performance targets (May *et al.*, 2007). The outcome was consistent with the 'net-widening' reported in South Australia, because there has not been any accompanying increase in reported rates of cannabis use in the general community. Self-reported cannabis use among the public aged 16–59 declined from between 10.3–10.8% in the 5 years prior to the change, to 9.7% in 2004–2005, 8.7% in 2005–2006 and 8.2% in 2006–2007 (Nicholas *et al.*, 2007: 43). Similarly, the proportion of 16 to 24 year olds who reported using cannabis in the last year has decreased from over 26% in the 5 years prior to reclassification to 25.3% in 2003–2004, 23.6% in 2004–2005, 21.4% in 2005–2006, 20.9% in 2006–2007 (Nicholas *et al.*, 2007: 44).

May and colleagues (2007) conducted an internet-based survey of 749 respondents in England and Wales between June and November 2005. Although the authors acknowledged that the sample could not be said to be representative of the general population, they found 77% supported the reclassification from B to C. With regards to knowledge of the change, 98% knew that cannabis remained illegal under the changes and 78% believed that they had a fairly good understanding of the changes, 74% understood that street warnings could be issued and 69% that the cannabis user could be arrested. However there was some confusion as to how juveniles (as against adults) were treated under the provisions, and many incorrectly thought that police 'turning a blind eye' to cannabis was legitimate under the reforms (May *et al.*, 2007). A small interview study of 61 young people between that ages of 14 and 21 who had either used cannabis or been stopped by police regarding drugs found that, while 69% supported reclassification to Class C, 52% did not understand that nothing had changed for those under 18 and they would still be arrested for cannabis possession. Interviews with 150 police officers indicated that 59% believed the government were wrong to reclassify cannabis as a Class C drug, and 93% of officers surveyed stated that they had come across people who believed – or more likely claimed to believe – that cannabis had been legalized (May *et al.*, 2007).

An analysis of cannabis seizure data from London and a number of other boroughs in the United Kingdom suggests that the potency of sinsemilla has increased from a mean of 6% THC in 1996 to 13% in 2005, and that increasingly in many boroughs sinsemilla dominates the market over resin (hash) and herbal cannabis (Potter *et al.*, 2008). However, these changes are not a result of reclassification, but rather reflect increased domestic cannabis production in the last 5–7 years (Personal communication May, 2007), primarily by hydroponic cultivation. Similar trends have been observed in a number of other countries around the world (United Nations Office of Drugs and Crime, 2006).

As mentioned in Chapter 2, trends in both cannabis-related drug treatment and mental health presentations in the United Kingdom since reclassification were examined in the UK Drug Policy Commission submission to the ACMD Cannabis Classification Review 2008 (UK Drug Policy Commission, 2008). They found that there had been increases in the number of people, particularly those under 18, in treatment for problematic cannabis use. Since reclassification, the number of hospital admissions for mental and behavioural disorders diagnosed as having been caused by cannabis use had also increased. They noted that, although these increases could be seen as concerning, this was not necessarily an indication that harmful use had increased. Rather, better detection of problem users or more treatment places could also explain the increase, particularly as indications were that rates of cannabis use had declined since reclassification. They noted that other economic, social, and cultural factors were likely to be stronger drivers of cannabis use than its classification status (UK Drug Policy Commission, 2008). In addition, there is typically a 5- to 10-year lag between initiation to cannabis use and presentation to treatment for problem use, so people presenting for treatment in the present probably initiated use five or more years ago.

Netherlands

Impacts on rates of use

The evaluation literature on the effect of the cannabis *coffee shop* system in the Netherlands has been controversial. In two publications, MacCoun and Reuter (1997; 2001b) compared available data on the effects of drug laws on cannabis use across the Netherlands, United States, Denmark, and Germany. In the second of these papers, the authors analysed data from 28 separate studies that employed adequate controls. They concluded that reductions in criminal penalties in the Netherlands from 1976 to 1992 had little effect on cannabis use, but they suggested that the increase in commercial access in the Netherlands from 1984 to 1992 with the growth in numbers of cannabis *coffee shops* (termed by them *de facto legalization*) was associated with growth in the cannabis-using population, including young people. For example, they claimed that lifetime prevalence of cannabis use among Dutch aged 18–20 increased consistently and sharply from 15% in 1984 to 44% in 1996, and that past-month prevalence in this group increased from 8.5% to 18.5% over the same period (MacCoun & Reuter, 2001b). They hypothesized that the rapid increase in cannabis use in the Netherlands in the mid-1980s *may have been* the consequence of the gradual progression from a system of passive *depenalization* to a *commercialization* era which, up until 1995 at least, allowed for greater access and increasing promotion of cannabis (MacCoun & Reuter, 2001b). This included indirect effects such as heightened salience and glamorization of cannabis because of visible promotion especially in counter-culture media advertising, and through postcards and posters (MacCoun & Reuter, 2001b). However, MacCoun and Reuter (2001b) note that the increases in prevalence in the Netherlands from 1992 to 1996 were similar to trends that occurred in Norway, the United States, the United Kingdom, and Canada. The latter points to the important role of poorly understood social and cultural influences on the prevalence of cannabis use. They also noted that, even with this more liberal policy, rates of cannabis use in the Netherlands were no greater than those in the United States, which had a consistently more punitive policy towards cannabis use over the same period.

MacCoun and Reuter's glamorization hypothesis has been criticized by others (e.g. Abraham *et al.*, 2001; de Zwart & van Laar, 2001; Korf, 2002). For example, Abraham and colleagues (2001) criticized the MacCoun and Reuter analysis for its comparison of data from cities with statistics for whole nations, and questioned the validity of some of the comparative data sets. Both points have been effectively rebutted by the authors (MacCoun & Reuter, 2001a; 2001b).

In a subsequent paper, Korf (2002) looked at trends in current, rather than lifetime, cannabis use and showed that, across the Netherlands, other European countries, and the United States, there had been wave-like trends in cannabis use. He noted that it was 'striking' that these trends in cannabis use among young people in the Netherlands mirrored the four stages in the availability of cannabis identified by MacCoun and Reuter (2001b). Thus, the number of cannabis users peaked in the 1960s and early 1970s, when cannabis distribution occurred through an underground market. Recent use of cannabis by Dutch youth increased during the 1970s, when house dealers were taking over from the underground market. It increased again during the 1980s, when *coffee shops* established themselves as the sale points for cannabis. In the late 1990s, rates of recent use among Dutch youth stabilized. Rates decreased by the end of the 1990s, after the age of access to coffee shops was increased from 16 to 18 years in 1996 and the number of coffee shops was reduced (Korf, 2002).

Korf (2002) concludes nonetheless that it is doubtful that changes in cannabis use were causally related to changes in cannabis policy. More recently, an analysis of the changes in cannabis prevalence among Dutch secondary students aged 12–17 found that these changes were paralleled by changes in the age of first use of cannabis. Average age of onset of cannabis use decreased from 15 years in 1992 to 14 years in 1996. After the legal age of buying cannabis from *coffee shops* was raised in 1996 the age of onset stabilized through to 2003 (Monshouwer *et al.*, 2005). However, as Korf (2002) noted, after raising the age limit in *coffee shops,* Dutch students were more likely to obtain their cannabis from outside *coffee shops*, mainly from friends. This could have increased the likelihood of them being offered other drugs or getting involved in other crime (Korf, 2002; Monshouwer *et al.*, 2005).

Impacts on patterns of use and market access

A project commenced by Peter Cohen, Craig Reinarman, Stephan Quensal, and Lorenz Bollinger has involved using a standardized survey instrument to compare representative samples of experienced cannabis users (used 25 times or more) in three cities with different cannabis policies. The surveys began in Amsterdam in 1995, Bremen in 1998, and San Francisco in 1999 (Borchers-Tempel & Kolte, 2002). The study found that the prevalence of different 'consumer types' varied across the cities. Thus 'moderate' users – long-term users of the drug who use regularly and tend to limit their use to reach a desired level of intoxication – were more prevalent in Amsterdam (19%) and Bremen (19%), but were less likely to be found in San Francisco (10%) (Borchers-Tempel & Kolte, 2002). Conversely, San Francisco had higher rates of 'leisure-oriented occasional consumers' (29%) and heavy (mostly dependent) users (22%). The study concluded that 'repressive policies do not reduce consumption, but do produce problematic consumption patterns among many of those who defy authority' (Borchers-Tempel & Kolte, 2002: 411). However, this conclusion seems to over-state the impact of policy on rates of use, and does not seem to entertain that there are likely to be other social and cultural differences between the three cities which were important.

Nonetheless, the work confirms that the Dutch have shown that a system of cannabis supply can be established which largely separates the cannabis market from that for other illicit and potentially more harmful substances. Some 87% of the Amsterdam sample said that they usually bought their cannabis from cannabis *coffee shops*, whereas more than 80% of the Bremen sample and 95% of the San Franciscan sample said they usually obtained their cannabis from friends who knew a dealer, or from 'known dealers'. Furthermore, 85% of the Amsterdam sample, compared to 51% of the Bremen sample and 49% of the San Francisco sample, said that no other drugs were available from the source where they obtained their cannabis (Borchers-Tempel & Kolte, 2002: 399–400).

A more recent paper from the same study comparing rates of use in Amsterdam and San Francisco found no evidence that 'criminalization' (in San Francisco) reduced use or that 'decriminalization' (in Amsterdam) increased use. Rather, except for higher rates of cannabis use in San Francisco, they found strong similarities across both cities (Reinarman *et al.*, 2004). In contrast to the conclusions of the Borches-Temple and Kolte (2002) paper, they concluded that regular cannabis users organized their use around sub-cultural norms about when, where, why, with whom, and how to use, rather than around laws and policies (Reinarman *et al.*, 2004).

Conclusions on Dutch policy

So what can we say about the impact of the Dutch cannabis policy on prevalence and patterns of cannabis use and harms? First, there is a consensus that depenalization in the Netherlands did not, in itself, lead to increases in population levels of cannabis use among adults nor among young people. This finding is consistent with results in Australia and the United States. Secondly, the Dutch system does appear to have successfully separated the market for cannabis from other substances. The majority of cannabis users who buy their cannabis from the regulated environment of *coffee shops* do not need to have contact with other illicit sources (dealers or friends who have contact with dealers), where they may be exposed to other drug use and criminality.

Thirdly, there are competing views of the impact of the 'commercialization' of cannabis sales from the mid-1980s to mid-1990s. On the one hand, the increases in prevalence of cannabis use among youth appear to mirror changes in other countries that began prior to this period. On the other hand, the prevalence changes correlate with changes in policy, increasing as access and availibility increased. On balance we would say that the case is still open about whether *de facto legalization* led to more use by youth and an earlier age of onset; it cannot be ruled out that increases in youth prevalence *may have* been associated with increasing *de facto* legalization, and subsequent decreases with tightening up of this policy. The critical point here is that, while international research shows that there is little relationship between rates of cannabis use and cannabis policy when use remains illegal in both a *de facto* and *de jure* sense, the Dutch experience raises the question about whether going beyond *depenalization* to *de facto legalization* may increase rates of cannabis use among the young, who are most vulnerable to the adverse effects of cannabis. Some will disagree with this analysis, but we believe at this stage a cautious conclusion is warranted, pending further research.

Italy

Changes in Italian policies towards cannabis and other drugs should ideally provide a perfect case to examine the impact of depenalization using an ABA type research design (penalization-depenalization-repenalization). The popular view is that there has not been any relationship between the legal changes and prevalence of cannabis (and other drug use). An often-cited paper by Solivetti concludes:

> The first and most impressive fact that emerges from the Italian history of drug policy is the lack of visible impact of the various legislative actions in this field. What is particularly impressive is the lack of visible impact as regards the – in most cases increasingly – repressive actions. The harsh and undifferentiating repressive sanctions of the 1950s did not prevent the drug diffusion boom of the 1960s. The increased criminal sanctions against drug traffickers, provided by the 1975 Act, did not result in curbing drug diffusion; on the contrary, the latter grew more and more. The reintroduction of sanctions against drug use in 1990 had no visible impact on the phenomenon.
>
> (Solivetti, 2001: 51)

One issue is that Solivetti only analysed data series on cannabis and other drug use up to 1998. Now, 10 years later, a longer data set should have accrued to investigate impacts of the last depenalization, which came into effect in Italy in 1993. The EMCDDA has noted that rates of cannabis use in a number of European countries including France, Spain, and Italy have increased in recent years and that they are developing methodologies to investigate more frequent (daily) use patterns, which are likely to be indicative of cannabis dependence and other harms (EMCDDA, 2007a). So, consistent with our conclusions for other countries, while there is no evidence supporting the view that cannabis depenalization in Italy resulted in increase rates of use and problems, it needs to be noted that further research would be useful to confirm the rather limited evidence examined to date.

Switzerland

As noted in the previous chapter, while the consumption of cannabis is prohibited by law in Switzerland, police forces in the 26 Swiss Cantons exercise considerable discretion in how the law is applied. Capitalizing on this and using data from the WHO European Health Behavior in School-Aged Children survey (HBSC) study, Schmid (2001) employed hierarchical linear modelling to examine the impact of peers, urbanization and the severity of enforcement of cannabis laws on rates of cannabis use among 3,107 15 year olds. The study suggested that while living in urban areas affected the extent to which cannabis use was affected by peers, whether the canton in which one lived had repressive or more lenient cannabis policy did not have any effect on cannabis use by individuals (Schmid, 2001).

Czech Republic

The Czech Republic provides a unique example of a substantial evaluation of the effects of a move to tighten laws, that is, to criminalize possession and use of cannabis (and of other drugs) where they had not been criminalized. The criminalization was passed in 1998 after sharp controversy and over the veto of President Vaclac Havel. In the aftermath the government commissioned a substantial evaluative study by a group of Czech experts, advised by US academics (Moravek, 2008). The evaluation tested with quantitative data several propositions about the effects of the introduction of penalties for the possession of illicit drugs for personal use. The propositions that 'availability of illicit drugs will decrease' and that the 'number of ... illicit drug users will decrease' or at least stabilize were rejected on the basis of the study, while a number of other hypotheses could not be reliably tested. Qualitative studies filled out the picture of the effects of the legislation, including no evidence of effects on 'drug scenes'. However, the new law provided the police with opportunities to pressure persons of interest for other reasons. One informant commented about this, 'I must admit it is not completely legal. In a way, it is a bit of blackmail' (Zabransky et al., 2001). While penalties for possession for personal use were only enforced randomly and occasionally in the two years after adoption of the legislation, there were substantial costs to the state from the legislation, without any apparent benefit (Zabransky et al., 2001).

Economic analyses

As noted, the Czech study included a 'cost and benefit analysis', which concluded that the penalization of possession for personal use was economically disadvantageous to the state in the short run, and probably also in the long run

(Zabransky *et al.*, 2001). In terms of moves away from criminal penalties, there have been at least four economic analyses of the impact of introducing *prohibition with civil penalty schemes* on law enforcement and other costs. Civil penalty schemes can in principle be far cheaper than criminal or diversion schemes in terms of enforcement and justice resources, because civil offences can usually be dealt with more expeditiously and with fewer procedural protections (Pacula *et al.*, 2005). For example, a recent analysis in Western Australia of the cost of dealing with a minor cannabis offence through the issuing of an infringement notice, versus dealing with it through the court system, found a 7:1 net cost benefit of infringement notices over court process-ing (Christie & Ali, 2000; Drug and Alcohol Office, 2007b), which mirrored the findings of an earlier study of the South Australian scheme (Brooks *et al.*, 1999). Economic analyses have found that the magnitude of potential criminal justice savings depends on the size of the jurisdiction, the cost of the existing mechanisms for control of minor cannabis offences, and the expiation rate achieved by the infringement notice schemes, with greater savings from higher expiation rates. Annual savings were estimated at $US100 million in California (Aldrich & Mikuriya, 1988), and at $US24.3 million in Massachusetts (Miron, 2002). In the much smaller polity of South Australia, the estimated savings were less than $US1 million (Brooks *et al.*, 1999). However, as Hall and Pacula (2003) have suggested, given the way the budget process in democracies works, it is not clear where these savings would in fact be directed – and doubtful that it would be towards such 'social dividends' as tackling more serious crime or otherwise reducing drug-related harm (Lenton, 2005).

Medical marijuana

Studies of the impact of introduction of medical marijuana schemes on rates of cannabis use in the general community are difficult to locate. While the US General Accounting office conducted a thorough investigation of such initia-tives in Oregon, Alasks, Hawaii, and California in 2002, this did not include impacts on rates of cannabis use generally (US House of Representatives United States General Accounting Office, 2002). Khatapoush and Hallfors (2004) analysed three waves of telephone survey data in 1995, 1997, and 1999 to investigate the impact of Proposition 215, the Compassionate Use Act, which came into effect in California in late 1996. They compared attitudes and use rates among 16 to 25 year olds in selected communities in California and 10 control states. They concluded that medical marijuana policy had little impact on youth and young adult marijuana-related attitudes and use in the selected communities in California and beyond. After Proposition 215 came into effect, Californians were less likely to see occasional marijuana use as risky, and were more approving of marijuana legalization and use for medicinal purposes, but were less approving of (recreational) marijuana use. Rates of recent cannabis use (past month and past year) were higher in California compared to control states, both before and after Proposition 215 came into effect.

Conclusions and implications

This chapter reviewed the available literature on the impact of cannabis reforms which have been undertaken within the provisions of the existing international drug treaties and conventions. It is apparent that only a minority of the examples of reform identified in the previous chapter have been subjected to any evaluation that can assess the impacts of the reforms on rates of cannabis use and cannabis-related harm.

Furthermore, two caveats need to be made. First, as we have done in this chapter, one needs to take into account that much of the research which has been conducted is compromised by methodological flaws. Secondly, caution also needs to be exercised in drawing conclusions from one reform example in one country and trying to implement similar changes in another. Geographical, social, cultural, political, legislative, and other contextual factors are likely to influence reforms and their impacts. Thus, it is important that any reforms which are implemented are subject to rigorous evaluation. Ideally the results of any such evaluations should allow the reforms to be modified to minimize any unintended adverse effects, such as net widening. Nevertheless, despite these caveats, the following conclusions can be drawn on the basis of the available literature.

Impacts on prevalence of use

There does not appear to have been any large increases in cannabis use in countries that have maintained the *de jure* illegality of cannabis but implemented reforms which, either at a national or subnational level, have reduced the penalties to civil or administrative sanctions. Among these policy reforms, the shift from strict prohibition to *prohibition with civil penalties* is the best researched. The methodologically stronger studies fail to find that these changes in penalties have large impacts on the prevalence of cannabis use at a population level or among school children. Although the results here may be limited by low statistical power and limited sample size to detect small increases, the available evidence suggests that if increases in use are found at the general population level, they are likely to be small.

The evidence on the impact of depenalization in the Netherlands suggests that it has not resulted in increased prevalence of cannabis use at a community level, and that it has been successful at separating the cannabis market from other drug markets. Questions remain open about the extent to which the increased commercialization of cannabis in the Netherlands in the period 1992–1996 may have resulted in more cannabis use by the young and in an earlier age of onset. If it did, then the age restrictions and other changes introduced in the *coffee shops* in the mid 1990s appear to have arrested this trend.

Regarding impacts of reforms on prevalence of cannabis use, it is also apparent from a number of the studies that, at least as long as the illegality of cannabis is maintained, the laws and sanctions which apply seem to have, at most, a relatively modest impact on rates of cannabis use. In a number of examples, trends in cannabis use appear to be independent of the penalties which apply. It is likely that, as far as reforms under the existing international treaties are concerned, other non-legal factors such as social, economic, and cultural trends, some of which exert their influence across state and national boundaries, have a far greater impact on cannabis use than the penalties which apply in a particular jurisdiction to that very small proportion of users who are ever arrested.

Reducing the adverse consequences of prohibition

The research suggests that those reforms which have been undertaken under the existing international drug conventions have reduced, but not eliminated, some of the adverse social impacts of prohibition on individuals. They also appear to reduce the costs to the criminal justice system of prosecuting cannabis use offences. However, these benefits can be undercut by police practices that increase the number of users who are penalized, or enforce the law in a discriminatory way. The costs to individuals apprehended can be substantially reduced by civil rather than criminal sanctions for many users. Nonetheless these schemes can have a disproportionate impact on those of limited financial means and the socially disadvantaged, who may still end up being processed by the criminal courts because they are unable to pay fines. Although savings in criminal justice resources have been noted and appear to be proportional to the size of the jurisdiction, it is unlikely that these savings are in practice strategically diverted to address other more serious crime problems, but rather 'disappear' into general police budgets or central revenue.

While there is debate about whether the *de facto* legalization system in parts of the Netherlands contributed to increasing rates of use, there is good evidence that the Dutch *coffee shop* system has removed the risk of legal penalties for most users and effectively separated the market for cannabis from other illicit drugs. It may be the case, however, that the age restrictions introduced in the *coffee shops* in the mid-1990s may have paradoxically increased adolescent exposure to the illicit market and thereby increased associated risks and harms.

Chapter 6

Beyond the current drug conventions

So far in this volume we have considered measures which have been taken within the context of the current international drug control regime. Now we turn our attention to measures which would in one way or another move beyond the limits of the regime.

Some such measures could be taken by concerted action by the parties to the current conventions, or by a substantial majority of them. Such measures would involve removing cannabis from the conventions, or fundamentally altering the provisions of the convention covering cannabis. For completeness, we list these alternative measures, but do not explore them in any detail. In the current global cultural politics of drugs, it seems unlikely that any of these measures could be successfully pursued.

Other measures could be taken by a single state or by a group of states. There is considerable variation between these measures in the extent to which they can be seen as politically viable at present. However, they are discussed in somewhat more detail, because possible paths forward seem more likely to be drawn from these alternatives. We also discuss some options for an alternative international cannabis regime to the present one.

Removing the coverage of cannabis in the conventions

The 1961 Convention (UN, 2007a) obliges parties to 'limit exclusively to medical and scientific purposes' the 'production, manufacture, export, import, distribution of, trade in, use and possession' of the substances covered by it (Art. 4, §1.c).

While cannabis is presently listed under Schedule I and IV of the treaty, this scheduling is not inscribed in the treaty itself, and it would theoretically be possible not only to shift cannabis to another schedule but to deschedule it altogether. The primary Article which refers specifically to cannabis, Article 28, requires that cannabis production be licensed and controlled, and that a state agency act as the buyer and wholesaler of the crop.

So long as cannabis is in Schedule I of the 1961 Convention, each party to the treaty is obliged to keep as 'punishable offences' production, trading in or possession of it (Art. 36), 'subject to its constitutional limitations'. This is further backed up by Article 3, §1 of the 1988 Convention (UN, 2007b), which requires parties to establish production, distribution, possession, or purchase of substances covered under the 1961 and 1971 Conventions 'as criminal offenses under its domestic law'.

In theory, then, there are three ways in which cannabis could be removed from the scope of the 1961 Convention:

1 By amendment under Article 47. This would require either unanimous consent, or the convening of a Conference of the parties by action of the Economic and Social Council (ECOSOC) of the United Nations. The official Commentary on the 1961 Convention points out that ECOSOC has the option to refuse to call an amending Conference, but that on the other hand the General Assembly of the UN could also take the initiative in amending the Convention (UN, 1973: 462–3).

2 By termination of the Convention as a result of a sufficient number of denunciations (withdrawals) from the Convention to reduce the number of parties below 40.

3 By removal of cannabis from any of the Convention's schedules. This would still leave in place Article 28, requiring state control and licensing of production and a state monopoly wholesaler. Such a 'modification', as it is termed by Andenas and Spivack (2003), must be based on the recommendation of a WHO Expert Committee, and would require a majority vote in the Commission on Narcotic Drugs (CND), and in the UN ECOSOC if any party appealed the CND decision.

None of these three methods of removing cannabis from the 1961 Convention seems likely to succeed in the foreseeable future, although it would be an interesting first step to try to delete cannabis from Schedule IV of the Convention. Accordingly, they will not be further considered here.

For completeness, we might mention a fourth way in which international control of cannabis could theoretically end. It has happened that international treaties simply fall into disuse as conditions change, without any formal termination or denunciation. 'It is, indeed, generally considered that a treaty falls into desuetude when its non-application by parties over a period of time establishes their consent to let it lapse' (Pauwelyn, 2003: 143). This is the case, for instance, with the two conventions which were adopted by the European colonial powers in 1889 and 1919 to control the market in spirits in Africa (Bruun et al., 1975). Again, this seems unlikely with respect to cannabis in the foreseeable future.

Actions by a single country or a group of countries

Reinterpretation

The INCB and other organs of the international drug control system put forward interpretations of the language of the conventions, and the INCB has been quite vociferous about its interpretations. But there is no interpretation of the language of the treaties which is binding on parties to them, and states have routinely adopted interpretations which differ from those of the INCB.

However, the room for manoeuvre on interpretations is in principle limited by the general rule in international law that words should be interpreted in terms of their plain meaning, and that 'pacta sunt servanda': as stated in Article 26 of the Vienna Convention on the Law of Treaties (UN, 2005a), which entered into force in 1980, 'every treaty … is binding upon the parties to it and must be performed by them in good faith'.

Beyond this, both the 1961 Convention (Art. 48) and the 1988 Convention (Art. 32) provide that in case of a dispute 'relating to the interpretation or application of this Convention' which cannot be settled by negotiation, mediation, or other means, it 'shall be referred to the International Court of Justice for decision'. The 1988 Convention specifies that any party to the dispute can make the referral. These provisions do not seem ever to have been invoked.

In view of the explicit and clear references to cannabis in the 1961 Convention, it would not be possible to credibly reinterpret the Convention as excluding it. With respect to the specific provisions bearing on cannabis in the 1961 and 1988 Conventions, there is much more scope for interpretation. As Krajewski (1999) notes, the conventions 'are formulated in a very broad, even vague manner', which 'allows for latitude in interpretation'. However, issues of interpretation fall primarily in the territory of alternative measures within the scope of the present international control system, dealt with in the preceding chapters. Accordingly, they are not further discussed here.

Denunciation

The 1961 treaty (UN, 2007a) provides a clear procedure for denouncing the Convention, that is, withdrawing from it with a specified notice period which amounts to less than a year (Art. 46). In the 1988 Convention (UN, 2007b) the specified notice period is one year (Art. 50). Helfer (2005: 1601) notes that 'the conventional wisdom holds that treaty exits are extremely rare events that governments undertake only after exhausting all other avenues of persuasion and influence'. However, compiling a database of ratifications and denunciations of treaties from 1945 to 2004, he found that exits were in fact not so rare; in that period there had been 1,547 denunciations or withdrawals, a little under

5% of the number of ratifications. Of the multilateral treaties that were concluded after 1945, 3.5% had been denounced at least once.

Denunciation of a treaty is on the one hand a legal action that removes a state's obligation to comply with the provisions of a treaty. On the other hand, it is also a public statement. As Helfer (2005: 1588) notes, 'withdrawing from an agreement (or threatening to withdraw) can give a denouncing state additional voice, either by increasing its leverage to reshape the treaty,… or by establishing a rival legal norm or institution together with other like-minded states'.

Leinwand (1971) puts forward an argument for an option of *selective denunciation* of the 1961 Convention, specifically with regard to cannabis. He considers the requirements generally considered in international law for separability of provisions in a treaty, and concludes that these requirements would be met in separating cannabis out. Leinward then justifies the selective denunciation in terms of the provisions for 'error' and 'fundamental change of circumstances' which are considered below. The end result of taking this path would be the same as full denunciation and reaccession with reservations, discussed next. Given that there is no provision for selective denunciation in the 1961 and 1988 treaties, taking this path might be less legally defensible than denunciation and reaccession with reservations.

It appears that no state has ever denounced any of the current international drug conventions.

Denunciation and reaccession with a reservation

Traditional practice has been that reservations to treaties can only be made at the time of accession to treaties. The 1961 Convention includes complex provisions on reservations, but the only provisions now applicable are in Article 50. Paragraph 2 provides for reservations with respect to 7 specific paragraphs of the treaty which are marginal to our present topic. Paragraph 3 provides that other reservations are only permitted if there are no objections or objections from less than one-third of the parties within 12 months after they have been notified.

The 1988 Convention does not include provisions on reservations, which means that the issue is governed by the Vienna Convention on the Law of Treaties between States 1969 (UN, 2005a:Articles 19–23). Though the provisions are somewhat complex, the effect is that a reservation will usually be permitted. In fact, both the Netherlands and Switzerland, in ratifying the 1988 Convention, made reservations against the application of some of the provisions on criminalization in Article 3.[17]

---

17 Switzerland's ratification in 2005 made these reservations: 'Switzerland does not consider itself bound by Article 3, paragraph 2 concerning the maintenance or adoption of criminal

There are recent precedents in international law for denouncing a treaty and immediately ratifying it with a reservation (Helfer, 2006). Thus in 1998 and 1999 Trinidad and Tobago and Guyana denounced their accession to the First Optional Protocol to the International Convenant on Civil and Political Rights and immediately reacceded with reservations blocking petitions concerning death penalty sentences to the UN Human Rights Committee. When the Committee made a ruling nullifying Trinidad and Tobago's reservation, Trinidad and Tobago again denounced the treaty. Guyana, however, has neither denounced the treaty nor withdrawn its reservation, while refusing to comply with the Committee's recommendations concerning capital punishment (Helfer, 2006: 372–3). In 2002, Sweden denounced the Convention on the Reduction of Multiple Nationality and Military Obligations in Cases of Multiple Nationality, and then reacceded with a reservation. However, Helfer (2006) also cites instances where governments contemplated or announced such actions and then refrained from acting because of concerns about reputational damage. This was the case, for instance, when the British Prime Minister initially proposed in 2003 to withdraw from the European Convention on Human Rights and then rejoin with a reservation (Helfer, 2006: 373).

Denunciation and reaccession with a reservation is thus a viable path for a state which wished to remove cannabis from its adherence to the 1961 Convention, though it would certainly draw adverse comment.[18] However, under present circumstances there might well be objection by one-third or more of the parties. In general in international law, objections to a reservation simply mean that there is no international agreement between the reserving state and the objecting state for the matters covered by the reservation, unless the objecting state is 'specifically denying the reserving party's status as a party' (Swaine, 2006: 319; UN, 2005a:Art. 21, §3). This would presumably pose no problem for a state reserving cannabis out of its obligations under the treaty. If at least one-third of the parties objected to reaccession at all, in objecting to the reservation, the reacceding and reserving state would presumably be excluded from the treaty – what Helfer (2006: 375) regards as an extreme case, and labels the 'nuclear option'. Under the wording of the 1961 Convention, if at least

offences under legislation on narcotic drugs.... Switzerland considers the provisions of Article 3, Paragraphs 6, 7 and 8 as binding only to the extent that they are compatible with Swiss criminal legislation and Swiss policy on criminal matters'. The Netherlands made a similar reservation with respect to Article 3, Paragraphs 6, 7, and 8.

[18] In fact, it was suggested as a path by Leinwand (1971: 424) in his early consideration of ways in which the United States could remove cannabis from its international commitments under the 1961 Convention.

one-third of the parties objected to the reservation but not to the reaccession, the reservation would not be 'permitted'. But it is not clear what would happen next.

The situation with respect to the 1988 Convention is clearer. A state could probably successfully remove its obligation to the more onerous requirement of criminalization of cannabis in the 1988 Convention by denouncing and then reacceding to that treaty, with a reservation.

Swaine (2006) reviews the situation in international law on objections to reservations and notes that objections are surprisingly uncommon, and those that are made are quite often untimely. Where there are objections to a reservation, it is rather unclear what their effect is; in fact, reservations generally appear to remain in effect, despite any objections to them.

It should be noted that another uncertainty concerning reservations is introduced by the fact that the 1961 and 1971 Conventions came into effect prior to the entry into force of the Vienna Convention on the Law of Treaties, which, as Swaine (2006: 308) notes, 'is formally limited to treaties concluded after the Convention itself came into force in 1980'. However, Swaine goes on to note, the Vienna Convention's provisions are 'often invoked under other circumstances'.

'Error' and 'fundamental change in circumstances' as grounds for withdrawing from a treaty or suspending its operation

Article 48 of the 1969 Vienna Convention on the Law of Treaties provides that an error which 'relates to a fact or situation which was assumed by that State to exist at the time when the treaty was concluded and formed an essential basis of its consent to be bound by that treaty' can be grounds for invalidating a state's consent to a treaty. Article 62 provides that 'a fundamental change of circumstances which has occurred with regard to those existing at the time of the conclusion of the treaty, and which was not foreseen by the parties', can be invoked as grounds for withdrawing from a treaty if 'the existence of those circumstances constituted an essential basis of the consent of the parties to be bound by the treaty; and the effect of the change is radically to transform the extent of obligations still to be performed under the treaty' (UN, 2005a). Such a change in circumstances can also be a ground for 'suspending the operation of the treaty'.

Leinwand (1971) considers the applicability of error in the case of cannabis and the 1961 treaty, concluding that 'the inclusion of cannabis in a narcotics treaty was a mistake ... in the state of scientific knowledge' at the time of the treaty's adoption. In terms of the development of knowledge since 1971, things are now less black-and-white than Leinwand's argument that cannabis is outside the ambit of 'addiction to narcotic drugs', but a strong argument can still be put forward in terms of degree of harm (see Chapter 2 above) that cannabis does not belong in the 1961 treaty. Leinwand (1971) also considers the applicability of the doctrine of 'fundamental change in circumstances', again primarily in terms of the change in knowledge since 1961. In the light of history, a parallel and perhaps stronger argument might be made about the radical change in the prevalence of use and social position of cannabis in a variety of societies since the early 1960s. In 1961, cannabis use was largely confined to some enclaves of entrenched traditional use in particular societies, and otherwise to small and marginalized fractions of the population. Almost a half-century later, the situation is quite transformed: in dozens of societies, cannabis use is widespread in youth populations, and is widely regarded as a normalized part of growing up. This could be seen as constituting a fundamental change in circumstances justifying withdrawal from or suspension of the application of the 1961 treaty to cannabis.

The 'error' and 'fundamental change of circumstances' provisions are of obvious significance for a treaty where there is no provision for denunciation. But both the 1961 and 1988 treaties, as noted, have such provisions, so in legal terms there seems little reason for invoking the arguments of error or a fundamental change in circumstances with respect to cannabis. Helfer (2005) notes that the doctrine of fundamental change in circumstances has largely fallen into disuse, in his view probably because of the general availability of the option to denounce.

On the other hand, any effort at change in obligations on cannabis under the international conventions is at least as much a political as a legal matter. In political terms, a state or state may well find it wise to add arguments of error and fundamental change in circumstances when a path of denunciation or denunciation followed by reaccession with reservation is being followed.

Post-ratification reservation

A potential alternative to denunciation and reaccession with a reservation is for a party which has ratified a treaty to later file a new reservation. Helfer (2006: 373) notes that 'late reservations have become a regular, if infrequent, component of modern treaty practice'. He continues that 'although legal commentators have frowned on this practice, it is sufficiently common that treaty depositories have developed different procedures for circulating late reservations to non-reserving states for their review'. The International Law Commission has recommended allowing such late reservations, but only if no other party objects within 12 months (http://untreaty.un.org/ilc/reports/

2001/2001report.htm; 2.3.1-2.3.3, p. 179). Such a rule would, of course, nullify a late reservation if a single party objected. However, this remains a recommendation, rather than a settled matter in international law.

Adoption of a new convention

One option for neutralizing the present international cannabis regime would be to adopt a new international treaty concerning cannabis. This could be a convention specifically about cannabis, or it could cover cannabis along with other topics – such as covering a broader range of substances. As Ku (2005a), an expert on the issue, states the traditional rule: 'There is tradition-ally a last in time rule for treaties, with the later in time treaty prevailing over the earlier in time one'. In practice, there is an 'implicit' denunciation 'when a new treaty on the same subject matter has been entered into' (de Matons, 2004).

These rules are clear when the two treaties are between the same parties. But it leaves open the question of what happens when a later treaty ratified by a smaller number of parties conflicts with an earlier treaty ratified by a larger number. The 1986 Vienna Convention on the Law of Treaties between States and International Organizations or between International Organizations (UN, 2005b) has provisions covering this circumstance. In this 1986 Convention, with respect to two states who are both parties to both treaties, 'the earlier treaty applies only to the extent that its provisions are compatible with those of the later treaty' (Art. 30, §§3, 4). When only one is party to the later treaty, the earlier treaty still governs 'their mutual rights and obligations'. However, this treaty has not been ratified by enough parties to be in force, so these rules are not clearly in effect.

The 1969 Vienna Convention (UN, 2005a) also has a relevant provision, concerning 'Agreements to modify multilateral treaties between certain of the parties only' (Article 41). The modification must not be prohibited by the earlier treaty, cannot affect 'the enjoyment by the other parties of their rights under the treaty or the performance of their obligations', and cannot involve a change 'incompatible with the effective execution of the object and purpose of the treaty as a whole'. In considering conflict between 'norms' (legal provi-sions) in different treaties, Pauwelyn (2003) discusses the situation where there are parties to the first treaty who are not party to the second. He draws on the distinction in discussions of international law between treaties imposing 'reciprocal' and those imposing 'integral' obligations (pp. 52–8). The 'reciprocal' type can be broken down conceptually into pairwise obligations between parties, while the 'integral' type reflects a higher common interest beyond pair-wise obligations. In the case of treaties of the 'integral' type, if the later treaty conflicts with the 'object and purpose' of the earlier treaty, Pauwelyn's view is that the earlier treaty takes priority (Pauwelyn, 2003: 306).

A further consideration in the relationship between an older treaty and a new treaty between a smaller group of states is the principle of 'lex specialis': that a more specialized treaty takes priority over a more general one (Pauwelyn, 2003: 384–416). By this principle, for instance, a treaty specifically on cannabis would take precedence over a treaty on a broader range of substances. In Pauwelyn's view, the provisions of Article 30 of the 1969 Vienna Convention giving priority to the later treaty take precedence over 'lex specialis' (Pauwelyn, 2003: 409). He offers no opinion on the relation between 'lex specialis' and Article 41.

The state of international law thus seems to be somewhat unsettled concerning the relation between an earlier general drug treaty ratified by a large number of states and a later more specific treaty signed by a subset of those ratifying the earlier treaty. It is clear that, despite the later treaty, states which ratify it still have obligations under the earlier treaty to states which did not ratify the second treaty. Whether the earlier or later treaty prevails for the obligations between states ratifying both treaties is likely to be a matter for dispute.

In terms of 'mutual rights and obligations', it is worth keeping in mind the specific nature of the international drug conventions. In part, the conventions are concerned with international matters, in particular with controlling both the legitimate and illegal trade in substances they cover. The provisions in the 1961 Convention requiring a government wholesale monopoly of the legitimate market (Art. 28), requiring authorizations for export and import (Art. 31, §4), and banning export to another nation except in accordance with that nation's laws and with an import license (Art. 31, §§ 1, 5) are clearly related to controlling international trade in a substance of public health significance, and could well be retained or adapted in a new convention. On the other hand, the 1961 and 1988 Conventions contain many provisions which do not specifically concern international trade, but have to do with a nation's own internal laws and regulations. It is in fact these requirements in the Conventions – the requirement that states limit use to 'medical and scientific medical purposes' (1961 Convention, Art. 4), the requirement that production sale and possession be criminalized (1988 Convention, Art. 3, §1), and so on – which would need to be changed if a country wished to move to a legal internal market in cannabis. So long as a new convention provided for control to be maintained with respect to exports, in particular to countries continuing under the full application of the 1961 and 1988 Conventions, there is a strong argument that the 'mutual rights and obligations' to other parties would be maintained.

On the other hand, ironically, the parts of the conventions dealing with internal markets and matters might well be seen as evidence that the treaties are 'integral' rather than 'reciprocal' in nature.

In Part III of the present volume, we offer for consideration a Draft Framework Convention on Cannabis Control as a concrete example of what a new convention might contain. It is to a considerable extent modelled on the Framework Convention on Tobacco Control, but, in line with the discussion above, retains in large part the provisions of the 1961 Convention dealing with international trade and markets.

Addition of cannabis to an existing convention

The same purpose of providing a last-in-time substitute for the 1961 and 1988 conventions with respect to cannabis might be served by adding cannabis to an existing international treaty. Spivack (2004) has suggested that cannabis might be added to the Framework Convention on Tobacco Control (WHO, 2005). This Convention has provisions for adding Annexes and Protocols (Arts. 29 and 33). However, the wording of the Convention throughout is in terms of tobacco, and cannabis could not conceivably be added to its scope without an Amendment. Amendments require a three-quarters vote of the parties, and then accession to the amendment by at least two-thirds before they go into force (Art. 28). Adoption of a new convention would probably be an easier process than amending the FCTC to include cannabis.

Passing conflicting domestic legislation

A method of nullifying an obligation in international law guaranteed to raise considerable controversy would be for a state simply to pass legislation conflicting with the 1961 and 1988 Conventions: for instance, to set up a domestic control regime which legalizes production and sale of cannabis for non-medical use. The American legal literature on this has focused on the legality of doing this in terms of US law. The discussion is divided between the 'internationalists' who would insist that international law takes precedence over national law, and what have been labelled in the US the 'new sovereigntists', who insist that national legislation can pre-empt the application of an international treaty (Ku, 2005b: 339). In the specific case of the United States, it is settled that, under the US constitution, treaties have the same standing as national legislation – no less, but also no more. In the case of conflict between a treaty and a national law, the 'last in time ' principle applies, so that the more recently adopted of the two is valid. The constitutional situation varies in other countries, though the US position is not unusual (Conforti, 1993: 41–4).

This US principle conflicts with a provision of the Vienna Convention on the Law of Treaties (UN, 2005a), which applies to all treaties entering in force after 1980 (i.e. the 1988 Convention, but not the 1961 Convention): 'a party may not invoke the provisions of its internal law as justification for its failure to perform a treaty'. The Vienna Convention's provision codifies longstanding thinking in international law. With respect to international law, passing domestic legislation which nullifies an obligation would simply be a breach of treaty obligations. But in countries with principles concerning the status of international law similar to those applying in the US, it would be possible to nullify international law concerning cannabis by a new legislative enactment, if the country was willing simply to be in breach of its treaty commitments.

In the special case of the European Union, which has many characteristics of an international government, the general principle which has been established is that European Union law takes precedence over national law. But even in this case the issue is not wholly settled in all EU countries, particularly with regard to national constitutional provisions (Kumm & Comella, 2004).

Constitutional provisions or decisions

As noted above, the provisions in the 1961 treaty requiring criminalization of production, trading, and possession are subject to the party's 'constitutional limitations'. However, the 1988 treaty includes this exception with regard to criminalization only for 'possession, purchase or cultivation ... for personal consumption' (Art. 3 §2), and not for production and trading (Art. 3 §1.a). A constitutional protection of some sort against criminalizing production and trading thus will not countermand criminalization, in terms of the language of the Conventions, in any state which has ratified the 1988 Convention without reservation. Such provisions or decisions would fit under the previous rubric, 'passing conflicting domestic legislation', particularly if the constitutional provision or decision came into effect after the effective date of the relevant Convention, but they would probably be construed as a breach of the 1988 Convention.

Likely paths forward

There are thus several paths forward which could be taken by a single country or a group of countries inclined to allow a controlled legal market in cannabis. The simplest, in countries with a constitutional system like that of the United States, would be to pass domestic legislation enabling this. Under the last in time principle, this would nullify international law with respect to national law and the domestic market. However, with respect to international obligations, this would be a breach of the treaties, and the state would have to be willing to bear this onus.

A second straightforward path would be to denounce the 1961 and 1988 Conventions. An alternative which is likely to be more politically viable would be to denounce and reaccede with reservations. There is a substantial chance of objections to the reservations, and with respect to the 1961 Convention there might in that case be a considerable aftermath of international jurisprudence about the effect of the objections. If the country persisted, the end result might be denunciation.

A more complex alternative would be to join with like-minded countries and to negotiate a new international convention specifically about cannabis (or about some broader range of substances). To the extent that the provisions of the new convention conflicted with the provisions of the 1961 and 1988 Conventions, the intention would be that it would replace them, although as we have suggested the international law on this is somewhat debatable. The new convention, however, would probably not apply with respect to 'mutual rights and obligations' with parties to the 1961 or 1988 Convention who do not ratify the new convention. But the argument that the provisions of the new Convention which applied to a country's domestic market and laws are out- side those mutual rights and obligations seems strong in substance, whether or not it is in law.

A new treaty? Some concrete considerations

Auspices

One consideration in negotiating a new international convention on cannabis would be the auspices under which it would be negotiated. There is in fact no necessity for the negotiations to be hosted by any particular entity. It was in response to a US invitation, for instance, that conferences were convened and the original Hague Opium Convention was negotiated. Given the controversy which would be likely to surround the effort to negotiate a new cannabis convention, the simplest path forward might well be to proceed with a negoti- ating conference convened by this older path of invitation from one or more interested nations.

However, in recent years it has been common practice to negotiate such agreements under the auspices of an intergovernmental agency. In the United Nations system, the international drug conventions are under the auspices of the Commission on Narcotic Drugs, which reports to the UN Economic and Social Council (ECOSOC). An obvious alternative would be to take the precedent of the Framework Convention on Tobacco Control, which was negotiated at the call of the World Health Assembly and under the auspices of the WHO (Room, 2006). There is a strong logic in proceeding with a parallel convention on cannabis under WHO auspices, and the Draft Framework Convention on Cannabis Control in Part III below is worded in this way. Another international convention which involves psychoactive substances, the International Convention against Doping in Sport, was negotiated under the auspices of the United Nations Education, Scientific and Cultural Organization (UNESCO). It has been signed and put out for ratification, but is not yet in effect.

Another option would be to follow the earlier path taken in sports doping, and work under the auspices of a regional intergovernmental body. In 1989, an Anti-Doping Convention was negotiated under the auspices of the Council of Europe (Council of Europe, 1989), coming into force in 1990. As the Council's website explains (http://www.coe.int/t/dc/files/themes/dopage/default_en.asp?), 'the Convention is an "open" convention, which means it can be adopted by countries which are not members of the Council of Europe as well as countries outside Europe', and indeed Australia, Canada, and Tunisia have ratified it.

In the more general drug field, the Parliamentary Assembly of the Council of Europe adopted a resolution on 3 October 2007, calling for 'a European convention promoting public health policy in the fight against drugs' (Council of Europe, 2007a). The content envisaged for the convention is particularly concerned with establishing a public health approach concerning treatment services and the social handling of drug users (Council of Europe, 2007b). It would be a stretch to include within the proposed convention a new international agreement on cannabis. However, whether the agreement took this form or the form of a separate convention, the Council of Europe's longstanding interest in the drugs field would make it one of the logical potential auspices for a new cannabis treaty.

Content

Like the drug conventions and the tobacco convention (Room, 2006), a new cannabis treaty could be expected to contain three kinds of provisions: for domestic measures to control the market, for cooperation on international control, and for the international management of the agreement and its provisions. These provisions may be mandatory or recommended. Many of the provisions in the tobacco convention are encouraged but optional, while the provisions in the drug conventions tend to be mandatory. With respect to domestic measures, a major consideration is whether the 1961 Convention's requirement of a government wholesale monopoly would be kept. Whether it was or not, it might be expected that a new cannabis treaty would require or strongly encourage measures requiring licensing of producers, wholesalers and retailers, as is common in the case of alcoholic beverages and pharmaceuticals. A state monopoly or licensing regime gives the state strong tools to control the market. In particular, the state can then effectively forbid market participants from participating in the export of cannabis products except as allowed by the state to which they would be exported.

Another internal matter which potentially reaches across state borders is advertising and commercial promotion of sales. It might be expected that the cannabis convention would follow the tobacco convention in requiring that advertising and other promotion and sponsorship be banned if constitutionally allowed.

Otherwise, with respect to domestic matters such as conditions of sale, taxation provisions, educational programmes, treatment provision, etc., the choice would be to follow the lead of the tobacco convention, and spell out a set of recommendations and encouragements in the treaty, or to leave these matters to be settled in the individual society.

With respect to cooperation in international control, a major issue to be settled would be how arrangements in the new treaty interact with those of the drug conventions. At least with respect to countries which had not signed the new convention, the drug treaties' requirements for such matters as export and import authorizations, export declarations, seizure of illicit goods, and mutual assistance in law enforcement would remain in effect. The simplest path might be to continue such provisions in effect also in the new treaty, perhaps with a provision that signatories can waive such matters as export and import author-izations between themselves by mutual agreement. From the perspective of countries outside the new treaty, presumably the most important requirement would be of comity: that the new treaty should not alter the requirement of the existing drug treaties banning export to a country remaining prohibitionist.

Given the international environment into which it would come, strong consideration should be given to including provisions in the new treaty for a secretariat charged with watching over the new treaty and assisting signatories in implementing it. A counterpart for cannabis control to the International Narcotics Control Board would serve as a focal point in constructing a more realistic international drug control regime for cannabis.

Conclusion

With any of the paths forward outlined above, the basic drawback is that there will be vociferous opposition from a number of quarters – from the INCB, from the United States, and from a number of other countries. The opposition will be couched in terms of the old idealized rhetoric about the need for solidarity among humankind to defeat a common scourge (Room, 1999). In practical terms, no country up till now has been willing to weather this storm and actually to denounce any of the conventions.

Any move forward has to face these political issues and develop its own framing in terms of such ideals and principles as human rights and liberties, proportionality, and the minimization of harm (see e.g. Bewley-Taylor, 2004). Along with this, as we have noted, it would be wise for a state or states which are moving outside the present conventions to give reassurances that they will continue a commitment to some aspects of the current regime – in particular to controls on international trade which maintain comity, the principle that other states' domestic arrangements, for instance of cannabis prohibition, will be honoured. There are two paths forward which clearly do this: (1) denunciation and immediate reaccession with reservations (or the simpler but more difficult path of a late, post-accession reservation); and (2) negotiation and ratification of a new treaty covering cannabis.

Chapter 7

Paths forward from the impasse

By an accident of history, cannabis was included in the international drug control regime that was constructed in the course of the twentieth century. The final step was a complete prohibition on cannabis use under the terms of the 1961 drug convention. In an irony of history, this was shortly before rates of use of cannabis in youth cultures of developed societies took off. What had been a minor drug with use confined to a few scattered milieux in the developing world, and to some raffish and bohemian circles in a few affluent countries, soon became a symbol and carrier of the rebellion of mainstream youth cultures seeking cultural as well as political change. In country after country, youthful use of cannabis and the attempts by authorities to suppress it became a symbolic arena in which the cultural–political struggles of the 1960s and 1970s were partly fought out. The symbolic battles faded with time, but in the meantime, experimentation with cannabis had become a rite of passage for a significant fraction of those in every youth cohort since then. A substantial fraction of cannabis users have gone on to frequent use for a few years, and some to longer term use. Rates of recent use have fluctuated in the last 40 years, but it can now be said with some confidence that cannabis is an enculturated drug, used particularly during the life stage of youthful exploration and emancipation, in a large number of rich countries.

Even before the 1961 Convention, many governments had prohibited the non-medical sale or use of cannabis. The Convention pushed this process along, although not always expeditiously; for instance, it was not until 1986, with the expiration of a 25-year moratorium for customary use under the 1961 Convention, that India reluctantly outlawed the sale of many (but not all) forms of cannabis. As the wave of youthful use in the 1960s and 1970s hit developed countries, national and subnational governments responded in diverse ways. Some tried to deter use with increased penalties and more aggressive arrest policies; some reduced or eliminated penalties to reduce the widespread disregard of the law; some tried both approaches in succession or in some combination. After an initial round of experimentation with legal changes, the situation settled down after the 1970s in many places. In recent years, there have been further experiments with legal changes. Changes in the direction of lessening penalties for use have been motivated by the goal of reducing the widespread criminalization of and disadvantaging of those youth who are caught up in the cannabis prohibition laws while behaving in a way that is now so routine and whose harms are usually so distant from the individual offence and offender that it would take an active imagination to think that criminal justice actions are warranted. Changes in the other direction, increasing penalties, have been motivated primarily by arguments that adverse health consequences of cannabis have been underestimated or are increasing, perhaps as the result of increased potency. It is fair to note that those advocating increased penalties never cite evidence that such penalties have in fact deterred use in the past.

The international drug control conventions have served as a limit on the outer boundary of policy initiatives on decriminalization and legalization. No country which acceded to the Conventions has ever withdrawn from them. To our knowledge, no national government has legalized the growing, processing, or wholesaling of cannabis, except in restricted circumstances as a medication. The Swiss authorities have moved in this direction at least twice, but so far it has proved politically impossible. No country has formally legalized retail sale, although the Netherlands has done so in a de-facto way, to the continuing displeasure and disapproval of its neighbours and the guardians of the international drug control system. Often policy initiatives on cannabis have been restrained by appeals to the international conventions. In the meantime, we have cited evidence that the international control system has become more rigid and impervious to change; there is frequent reference to the argument that any relaxation of the status quo would 'send the wrong message'.

As it currently exists, the international cannabis prohibition regime by its nature and functioning imposes substantial personal and social harms. At the personal level, criminal and other penalties for those who are caught participating in the cannabis market often impose a heavy burden, not only on those caught but also on those close to them. This is obviously true for those who are punished for participating in the commercial production and distribution of cannabis. In some areas, such as parts of rural Canada and Morocco, a quite substantial part of the population is involved in cannabis production and thus is at risk of substantial personal harms. The burdens on the much broader group who are punished for possession or use of cannabis are also sometimes substantial. Very few people arrested for cannabis possession in the United States are sentenced to jail for that offence, but many of them will in fact spend time in jail during the pre-trial procedures. The comparisons in the Australian studies of the effects of depenalization show convincingly the broad range of adverse effects on the user and the family of convictions for cannabis possession or use.

Recent trends show increases in arrests for cannabis possession or use in many jurisdictions. The causes of this increase are not well understood because use has been stable or even declining in many of the same countries, but, by their nature, such arrests increase the adverse effects of policy at the personal level. Even in jurisdictions which have moved to mitigate the effects of arrest, there has been, to a greater or lesser extent, what criminologists call 'net-widening': more people have been caught up in the enforcement net, even if they suffer less serious consequences on average. At a personal level, the trend seems to be an increase in the adverse effects of prohibition in the face of steady or declining use, but without any indication that it is these increasing adverse effects that are driving down prevalence rates.

At a societal level, the illegality of the cannabis market imposes substantial adverse effects in a number of countries. It is often argued that widespread disregard of a particular law such as the prohibitions on cannabis creates disrespect for the law more generally. This is a plausible conjecture that remains to be tested. A law which criminalizes a profitable market linked with consensual behaviours, when widely flouted, often becomes a focus for official and police corruption. Impressionistically, there seems to be an upward trend also in these adverse effects at the societal level.

A half-century after the adoption of the 1961 Convention, and 40 years on from the initial rise in global cannabis use, it is time for policymakers to re-examine the status quo on control of cannabis and the premises on which the policy rests. What we have tried to assemble in this book is evidence and knowledge which would helpful to anyone prepared to undertake such a re-examination.

On the question of adverse health effects of cannabis, our review shows that the evidence base has become stronger in recent years. There are clear health harms from cannabis use. A driver who is high on cannabis is at increased risk of a traffic crash. Smoking cannabis probably increases the risk of respiratory disorders. Regular users risk developing dependence on the drug – difficulty in cutting down or quitting. Among the complex interactions between cannabis use and mental disorders, cannabis use seems to increase the risk of showing psychotic symptoms, but the population effects are small.

Clearly, in some markets the cannabis sold has become stronger in terms of THC content in recent years. For a naïve user, this may be problematic, although cannabis users are extremely unlikely to die of overdose. For a smoker who is seeking a particular state of intoxication, and titrates the dose accordingly, some have argued that stronger cannabis is actually less harmful to health, since the intake of potentially noxious combustion products is reduced. More rigorous assessments are needed of the causes and consequences of increased THC content.

The health harms from cannabis are clearly sufficient to justify substantial regulation on its marketing and availability. And it is important that the risks of health harms from cannabis use are communicated to users. On the other hand, public policy should take into account the relative risks in comparison to other common behaviours that carry some risk. In this comparative context the risks are on the low side. For instance, the health harms associated with both tobacco and alcohol use are clearly greater than those associated with cannabis.

Our analyses considered the available evidence on the effects of criminal regimes on cannabis use and problems. At the level of criminalization of production and wholesaling, there is little evidence on the effects of changes in laws, since there has been little experimentation (i.e. change in statutes) in this area in recent decades. However, it is clear that the prohibition of cannabis production and marketing, accompanied by moderately intrusive enforcement, has not succeeded in destroying the market. In fact, markets for cannabis flourish in all regions of the world, and particularly in more affluent countries. The fact that the transactions are often imbedded in social networks reduces the harms arising from the markets themselves, but this also points to the great difficulty in suppressing these markets in a democratic society which wishes to keep government intrusion to a minimum.

At the level of criminalization of use and possession, there is considerable evidence from a variety of legal changes aiming to ameliorate adverse effects of a regime of fully criminalized use and possession. Fairly consistently, the finding has been that changes in penalties for use have little effect on rates of use, or on problems arising from effects of the drug. In general, the attempt at deterrence of use or possession through criminal laws has failed to deter use, although it may somewhat affect the frequency and duration of use.

The findings in this area carry immediate implications for policy. A major consideration in debating proposed changes in cannabis use and possession laws is often the issue of 'the message it will send' to take some particular action.

'Sending the wrong message' can be interpreted in two quite different ways. One is instrumental; the message will be read correctly, so that cannabis use increases. That can in principle be tested, and we have cited above the lack of evidence that changes in criminal status has more than at most a small effect on use rates or intensity. The second interpretation is expressive; one duty of the government is to identify the appropriate behaviours, even if the label has no consequence. The old criminal laws against suicide, now mostly repealed, might be seen in that light. The second interpretation obviously is then not one subject to empirical test. But it is subject to considerations of ethics and human rights – the same kinds of considerations which led to the decriminalization of suicide. It is also appropriately subject to a balance test: does criminalization of a behaviour widely engaged in undercut the overall rule of law?

In terms of instrumental effects, the policy impact literature suggests that politicians should stop worrying about 'sending the wrong message'. Their actions in this area seem to have little effect on the behaviour in question. By contrast, their actions can certainly affect the adverse social consequences arising from the law and its enforcement.

In our report, we considered the options for moving beyond the status quo. A number of options have been implemented in one or another jurisdiction for depenalizing or otherwise reducing the adverse effects of criminalization of use and possession. In several cases the effects of these measures have been evaluated. It is clear that removing penalties for use and possession from the criminal law, and reducing them to a minimum, can have beneficial effects in reducing the adverse effects of criminal penalties on the user and those close to the user. But there is also a clear warning in the evaluation studies that, if such measures retain penalties for use and make it easier for police to enforce them, the result can be 'net widening', that is, an increasing number of persons, particularly the more disadvantaged, become caught up in legal enforcement systems.

As we have noted, the evidence from these evaluation studies is that removing or reducing penalties for use or possession appears to have little effect on rates of use. Reducing use and possession penalties to a minimum, without creating a situation which encourages enthusiastic police enforcement of the reduced penalties, thus seems a minimum step forward towards more rational cannabis policies.

A further step forward which some argue still stays within the regime of the Conventions is exemplified by the Dutch 'coffee shop' system. This de-facto legalizes use and possession, and indeed retail sale, under carefully controlled conditions. However, this option does not solve the 'back-door' problem, the fact that production and supply to the coffee shops remains formally illegal. This has probably diminished the attractiveness of this solution to other countries. An option which has not been explored is whether the systems of state-sanctioned cannabis shops in India offer any models for application elsewhere.

The other policy options which we have explored involve moving beyond the constraints of the existing Conventions. There are two primary ways in which this can be done. A state can simply denounce (i.e. withdraw from) the Conventions with respect to cannabis. The most likely way to do this for cannabis alone, without disturbing the state's adherence to the Conventions for other drugs, would be to withdraw from the 1961 Convention, and immediately reaccede to it with cannabis-specific reservations. As we have discussed, this path is not without potential brambles along the way, but is probably the most efficient and least politically problematic way of a state acting alone to move to handling cannabis production and sale with a system of regulatory controls.

The second possible way is for a like-minded group of states to adopt a new convention on cannabis control. Again, there are potential brambles, but generally the rule of a later treaty taking precedence over an earlier one would apply to the dealings of states that adopted the new convention with each other and in their internal markets. The states adopting the new convention would be spared the onus of withdrawing from the 1961 Convention, although they would continue to have obligations under the 1961 Convention concerning their dealings with states which stayed outside the new convention, for instance by controls on trade with those states.

Fifty years after the adoption of an unequivocal international prohibition on cannabis in the Single Convention on Narcotic Drugs, we face a very different world. The set of international rules and norms which were adopted then have not proven effective in the modern world, and they have adverse consequences for those who get caught up in their provisions. Effectively the conventions restrict the ability of signatory countries to adopt cannabis policies and laws which are driven by evidence. Further, in doing so they also restrict the accumulation of evidence to inform the development of new systems of control which may be more appropriate to the modern world. There is a clear need for change, and yet the international drug control system seems increasingly paralyzed and immobile. There is no question that moving forward will be difficult. But it is not impossible. In this report, our aim has been to draw on the available evidence to offer some possible paths forward.

Part II

Conclusions and recommendations of the Cannabis Commission

The Beckley Foundation Global Cannabis Commission

Benedikt Fischer, Faculty of Health Sciences, Simon Fraser University, Vancouver

Wayne Hall, University of Queensland

Simon Lenton, National Drug Research Institute, Curtin University of Technology, Perth

Peter Reuter, University of Maryland

Robin Room, University of Melbourne and Turning Point Alcohol & Drug Centre

Amanda Feilding, The Beckley Foundation

Conclusions about cannabis use and harms

1 In the last half century recreational use of cannabis has become widely established among teenagers and young adults in a broad range of developed countries and in some developing countries. In developed countries with the longest history of use, a substantial minority of users continue their use into middle age and beyond.

2 There are a number of health harms from smoking cannabis. Cannabis use impairs functioning in exacting tasks, and use before driving probably increases the risk of a traffic crash. About 10% of those who try cannabis develop dependence on the drug, and they have a somewhat higher risk of respiratory disorders, of impaired cognitive functioning (at least in the short term), and of developing psychotic symptoms or a psychotic disorder. Early and heavy use by adolescents may increase the risks of poor educational and other psychosocial outcomes in young adulthood.

3 The probability and scale of harm among heavy cannabis users is modest compared with that caused by many other psychoactive substances, both legal and illegal, in common use, namely, alcohol, tobacco, amphetamines, cocaine, and heroin.

4 Recently, concerns have been expressed about increased potency of cannabis products. Average THC content in many countries probably has increased, and the THC:CBD balance may have deteriorated (see p. 40), at least in part because of the illegality of cannabis production. The health consequences of any increases in THC content will depend on the extent to which users can titrate the dose of THC.

5 There are variations over time in rates of cannabis use within and between countries, but these variations do not seem to be affected much by the probability of arrest or penalties for use or sale, however draconian. The widespread pattern of cannabis use indicates that many people gain pleasure and therapeutic or other benefits from use.

6 It is probable that cannabis users who drive while intoxicated can harm others. Measuring tools are now available to establish whether a driver is under the influence of cannabis, and regulations and enforcement to deter this behaviour should be broadly implemented. Certain other harms to people from cannabis use are less well established. Role-failures from cannabis dependence (in work and family life) are probably the most important.

Conclusions about the effects of current policies

7 There have been longstanding efforts to deter cannabis use by prohibition and policing. Enforcement efforts in most countries have focused on the

arrest of users. In developed countries with large cannabis-using populations, the criminal penalties actually imposed for possession and use are usually modest by comparison with those possible by law. Moreover the probability of being arrested for any one incident of cannabis use is in the order of less than one in one thousand. The enforcement effort has not had much success in deterring use.

8 The rationale for severe penalties for possession offences is weak on both normative and practical grounds. In many developed countries a majority of adults born in the past half-century have used cannabis. Control regimes that criminalize users are intrusive on privacy, socially divisive, and expensive. Thus it is worth considering alternatives.

9 In addition to the substantial government resources expended in enforcing a prohibition regime, such a regime imposes very large secondary costs and suffering at the personal level. For example, a criminal conviction for cannabis possession can exclude an individual from certain jobs and activities, and arrest can impose personal and family humiliation. In countries where data are available, arrest rates are sharply higher for many minority and socially disadvantaged groups.

10 Measures to reduce penalties or to decriminalize possession and use have been adopted in numerous jurisdictions without an upsurge in use. Moreover these reform measures have had some success in ameliorating the adverse consequences of prohibition. However, the benefits of decriminalization can be undercut by police practices which may increase the number of users penalized, or by discriminatory enforcement of the law.

Beyond the international treaties

11 The present international treaties have inhibited depenalization and prevented more thoroughgoing reforms of national cannabis regimes. Regimes which do go beyond depenalization or decriminalization have been characterized by inconsistencies and paradoxes. For example, the Dutch coffee shops may sell cannabis products through the front door, but are not supposed to buy their supplies at the back door.

12 'That which is prohibited cannot easily be regulated'. There are thus advantages for governments in moving towards a regime of regulated legal availability under strict controls, using the variety of mechanisms available to regulate a legal market, such as taxation, availability controls, minimum legal age for use and purchase, labelling and potency limits. Another alternative, which minimizes the risk of promoting cannabis use, is to allow only small-scale cannabis production for one's own use or gifts to others.

13 There are four main choices for a government seeking to make cannabis available in a regulated market in the context of the international conventions:

    (1) In some countries (those that follow the expediency principle), it is possible to meet the letter of the international conventions while allowing *de facto* legal access. The Dutch model is an example.

14 If a nation is unwilling to do this, there are three routes which are the most feasible:

    (2) Opting for a *de jure* regulated availability regime which frankly ignores the conventions. A government that follows this route must be prepared to withstand substantial international pressure.

    (3) Denouncing the 1961 and 1988 conventions, and reacceding with reservations with respect to cannabis.

    (4) Along with other willing countries, negotiating a new cannabis convention on a supra-national basis.

15 The record is mixed concerning whether making cannabis use and sale legal in a highly regulated market would lead to increased harm from cannabis use in the long run. Experience with control regimes for other psychoactive substances teaches that lax regimes and allowing extensive commercial promotion can result in high levels of use and of harm, while stringent control regimes can hold down levels of use and of harm.

16 A nation wishing to make cannabis use and sale legal in a regulated market should draw on the substantial experience with other relevant control regimes for psychoactive substances. These include pharmacy and prescription regimes, alcohol sales monopolies, labelling and licensing, availability and taxation controls. Special attention should be paid to limiting the influence and promotion of use by commercial interests. Attention should also be paid to the negative lessons from the minimal market controls which have often applied for tobacco and alcohol, as well as to the positive examples.

Principles for policy analysis

17 Our policy recommendations below are guided by general ethical principles of public health action: measures to reduce harm should be proportional to the harm they aim to prevent, they should as far as possible have positive consequences and avoid negative ones, they should minimize effects on individual autonomy and they should be fairly enforced, particularly with regard to the less powerful or more marginalized groups.

18 Current cannabis policies may do some good, but there is a dearth of evidence in support of that claim. They clearly do harm to the many individuals who are arrested, they abridge individual autonomy and they are often applied unjustly. The enforcement of cannabis prohibition is also costly. The task is to devise policies that do better, taking all these aspects into account. We recognize the importance of the constraints imposed on policy by popular opinion, which usually supports a retention of prohibition.

19 The principal aim of a cannabis control system should be to minimize any harms from cannabis use. In our view this means grudgingly allowing use and attempting to channel such use into less harmful patterns (e.g. by delaying onset of use until early adulthood, encouraging all users to avoid substantial daily use, driving a car after using, and smoking cannabis mixed with tobacco).

Policy recommendations

20 Making policy recommendations involves value judgments and assessments of uncertainties. We offer our own recommendations for what constitutes good policy towards cannabis, recognizing that reasonable people can differ on the relevant values and in their assessments of contingencies.

Actions inside the box of the current international control regime

21 Under the current international control regime, the cannabis policy options available to governments are arguably limited to varying the severity of penalties for use. Given that more than minimal enforcement of prohibitions seems to do little to reduce use, the principal policy concern should be to minimize the adverse consequences of prohibition.

22 If a nation chooses to use the criminal law for controlling cannabis use, there is no justification for incarcerating an individual for a cannabis possession or use offence, nor for creating a criminal conviction. Retaining a criminal law on possession on the books as a handy tool for discretionary police use tends to result in discriminatory application of the law against the disadvantaged. Police should give very low priority to enforcing laws against cannabis use or possession.

23 A better option, the acceptability of which is more questionable under the international conventions, is to process violations administratively outside the criminal justice system. Fines should be low, and alternative sanctions such as referral to education or counselling should not be onerous, reflecting the proportionality principle.

Setting the international conventions aside

24 The international drug control regime should be changed to allow a state to adopt, implement and evaluate its own cannabis regime within its borders. This would require changes in the existing conventions, or the adoption of a new pre-emptive convention.

25 In the absence of such changes, a state can act on its own by denouncing the conventions and reacceding with reservations, or by simply ignoring at least some provisions of the conventions.

26 Any regime which makes cannabis legally available should involve state licensing or state operation of entities producing, wholesaling, and retailing the drug (as is true in many jurisdictions for alcoholic beverages). The state should, either directly or through regulation, control potency and quality, assure reasonably high prices and control access and availability in general and particularly to youth.

27 The state should ensure that appropriate information is available and actively conveyed to users about the harms of cannabis use. Advertising and promotion should be banned or stringently limited to the extent possible.

28 The impacts of any changes, including any unintended adverse effects, should be closely monitored, and there should be the possibility for prompt and considered revision if the policy increased harm.

Annex to Parts I and II: Research priorities

In preparing this volume, we found that the evidence available was often far less than we would have liked, even for developed countries with substantial research traditions. We lay out some of these research needs here.

We need to know more about the health effects of cannabis, about patterns of use and problems, and about the costs and effectiveness of different polices for attempting to discourage its use. Among the priorities for research on its health effects are the following:

- better epidemiological evaluations of the role played by cannabis use in motor vehicle crashes;
- longitudinal studies of the possible long-term health effects of continuing to use cannabis into middle age, especially its effects on the risks of cardio-vascular, respiratory disease, and cancer risk;
- research into the individual differences, particularly genetic, that underlie people's different reactions to cannabis in order to identify those with a susceptibility to experiencing extreme anxiety or psychosis;
- the effects of chronic cannabis use on the immune system and reproductive function in adolescence and young adulthood;
- the effects of cannabis use on risks of developing or exacerbating mental disorders in adolescence and young adulthood;
- the effects of regular cannabis use on cognitive and brain functioning in young adults;
- research into the perceived benefits of cannabis and into why the drug is so widely used;
- research on patterns and prevalence of cannabis consumption, and on wider social attitudes and behaviour, such as the attitudes of cannabis users towards the police and authority;
- research into the efficacy of various proposed medical applications for cannabis, particularly its potential as a painkiller, and further research into

the psychological and physiological effects of the 60+ naturally occurring cannabinoids found within cannabis;

Among the priorities for research on policies towards cannabis are the following:

- evaluations of the effectiveness of media campaigns and roadside drug-testing in reducing the contribution of cannabis use to the risks of motor vehicle crashes;
- evaluations of existing methods for discouraging early and regular cannabis use in adolescents and the development of more effective ways of discouraging such use;
- research into providing better assistance to cannabis users who develop problems related to their cannabis use and who wish to stop;
- research into the effects of different methods of discouraging illegal production and markets in cannabis;
- research into the effects of different systems of penalizing cannabis use and possession; research into the effects of *de facto* legal cannabis markets on patterns of cannabis use among adolescents and young adults;
- research into the effects of controls (price, availability, age restrictions, prescription regimes, etc.) in legal or quasi-legal markets on cannabis use and problems.

Part III

Draft Framework Convention on Cannabis Control

Background

Cannabis is subject to international control by the 1961 Single Convention on Narcotic Drugs, as amended in 1972 (http://www.incb.org/incb/convention_1961.html), and it is also affected by the 1988 Convention against Illicit Traffic in Narcotic Drugs and Psychotropic Substances (http://www.incb.org/incb/convention_1988.html). Because a basic principle of these conventions is that legitimate use of substances covered by them should be limited to medical and scientific purposes, they have been an effective block to efforts at a national or subnational level to move in any way to a regulatory system of control that aims to regulate use so as to minimize social and health harm.

While in principle these Conventions can be amended, this is not a practical possibility at the present time. An alternative path is for like-minded states to adopt a new Convention specifically devoted to cannabis. On the legal principle of 'last in time' taking precedence, this can be argued to take precedence in and between those states adopting such a new convention (see Chapter 6 above).

A precedent for a new convention covering a single psychoactive substance is the Framework Convention on Tobacco Control (FCTC; http://www.who.int/fctc/text_download/en/index.html). This convention was negotiated under WHO auspices, was adopted in 2003, and came into force in 2005. It has been proposed that cannabis might be added to this Convention (Spivack, 2004), but this would require an amendment process which is also not presently a practical possibility. The alternative, which is explored here, is to adopt a new convention, which might well be modelled on the tobacco convention.

Adapting the tobacco convention as a model

Comparative studies of the dangerousness of drugs are in substantial consensus that cannabis is less harmful to health than tobacco (see Chapter 2 above). By this criterion, modelling a new cannabis convention of the FCTC can be seen as a relatively conservative option. However, the FCTC is not as strong as public health advocates would wish. A major area of weakness is in terms of its lack of measures to monitor and control the international legal trade. This is an area in which the 1961 Single Convention is strong, reflecting a half-century of experience already at that time in regulating the legal trade in opiates and other medications. These provisions of the 1961 Single Convention would remain in force for any trade involving countries which remained outside a new cannabis Convention. It therefore seems prudent (and less confusing) to adopt the same provisions on international legitimate trade as in the 1961 Single Convention. Accordingly, these provisions are included in the proposed Convention, although their level of detail might seem at times excessive.

The model of the FCTC has also been strengthened in two other respects. The draft Cannabis Convention provides that it takes precedence over free trade and equal-treatment provisions of WTO and other trade agreements. This issue was omitted from the FCTC since no agreement satisfactory to public health could be reached on it. The draft Cannabis Convention also includes provisions concerning control of on-premise sales and consumption, drawing on experience from the alcohol field. However, the draft Cannabis Convention omits some wording from the FCTC that arose from the particularly iniquitous and duplicitous history of tobacco industry interference in science and policy, and the understandable special emphasis in the FCTC on tobacco smoke and emissions.

Notes on sources and adaptations in the draft convention

When it stated below that the draft uses another treaty's language 'unchanged', substitutions such as 'cannabis' for 'tobacco' will have been made. The following Articles are essentially unchanged from the FCTC, or have only minor adaptations, and are not commented on here: 2, 5–7, 11–13, 15, 17–38.

Preamble: Modelled on the preamble in the Tobacco Convention, but trimmed down.

Art. 1 – Use of terms: adapted from the FCTC largely unchanged, with an additional definition (h) for 'cannabis for personal use'. Note that the definition of 'cannabis products', as for 'tobacco products', is in terms of their intended use for human consumption (phrased slightly more widely for cannabis than in the FCTC). An alternative would be a definition in terms of psychoactive content, but this would be difficult to enforce. Note also Article 3 (2), taken from the 1961 Convention, specifically excludes from the draft Convention cannabis grown for industrial or horticultural use.

Art. 3 – Objective: restated in terms appropriate for cannabis: (a) supporting provision for legal non-medical use in States which allow this; (b) supporting prohibition in States which do not. Paragraphs 2 and 3 are taken from Paragraphs 2 and 3 of Article 28 of the 1961 Single Convention, except 'or misuse of' is omitted from the latter.

Art. 4 – Guiding principles: Slimmed down a little from the FCTC, dropping tobacco-specific provisions on liability and on economic assistance for displaced growers and workers.

Art. 8 – Regulation of production and sale: Replaces 'Protection from exposure to tobacco smoke' in the FCTC.

Article 28 of the 1961 Single Convention, on Cannabis control, applies Article 23 (written concerning opium) to cannabis. Accordingly, Paragraph 1 here is taken from Article 23, Paragraph 1 of the 1961 Single Convention.

Paragraph 2 is a new provision exempting 'cannabis for personal use' from Paragraphs 3 and 4.

Paragraphs 3 and 4 are from Article 23, Paragraph 2 of the 1961 Single Convention. The 1961 Convention provision that the state Agency must serve as the crop wholesaler is softened by allowing licensed wholesalers or manufacturers to receive the crop.

Paragraph 5 is from Article 19 of the 1961 Single Convention.

Paragraph 6 is from Article 30 of the 1961 Single Convention, adding provisions taken from experience with alcohol control for on-premise licenses and for controls of hours and days of sale, and for effective enforcement backed up by the threat of license suspension or loss.

Art. 9 – Sales to minors: this is from Article 16 of the FCTC, dropping the provision on sale of cigarettes 'individually or in small packets', and providing for a total ban on cannabis vending machines.

Art. 10 – Regulation of contents and disclosures: this is taken unchanged from Articles 9 and 10 of the FCTC.

Art. 14 – Demand reduction measures: 'limitation of use' is added to the FCTC text on 'cessation'.

Art. 16 – Provisions relating to international trade: Paragraphs 1–15 of Article 16 here, in all their excruciating detail, are taken from Article 31 of the 1961 Single Convention, except that 'form of the cannabis product' is substituted for the provisions on listing the name of the drug. Paragraph 16 is added, stating the precedence of the draft convention over any treaty which 'provides for free movement or equitable treatment of goods or services in trade or commerce'. The adequacy for its purpose of the language of this paragraph should be checked.

Adopting the draft convention

In principle, any state can call a conference of parties to negotiate a new treaty – it was at the call of the United States that the original Hague Opium Convention was negotiated. However, modern practice has usually been for an inter-governmental agency – regional or global – to auspice treaty negotiations. Thus the WHO was the convening body for the Framework Convention on Tobacco Control, and it will be seen that some provisions in the draft convention assume WHO auspices, since they are unchanged from the FCTC. Another intergovernmental body which has served as the convenor for a convention in the drug field is the Council of Europe, under which an Anti-Doping Convention was negotiated which eventually included signatory states from outside Europe, and which is presently considering a 'European convention promoting public health policy in the fight against drugs' (Council of Europe, 2007b).

Further discussion of considerations in adopting a new convention on cannabis can be found in Chapter 6.

Draft Framework Convention on Cannabis Control

Preamble

The Parties to this Convention,

Determined to give priority to their right to protect public health,

Recognizing that the control of the market for psychoactive cannabis products is a global issue with serious consequences for public health, calling for a comprehensive international response,

Reflecting the concern of the international community about the health and social consequences of cannabis consumption,

Concerned about the extent of worldwide consumption and production of cannabis products, as well as about the burden this places on families and on national health systems,

Recognizing that scientific evidence has established health and safety risks associated with the use of cannabis, including, but not limited to, its use by smoking,

Recognizing also that cannabis dependence is separately classified as a disorder in major international classifications of diseases, and that regular users of cannabis may become dependent,

Deeply concerned about smoking and other forms of cannabis consumption by children and adolescents worldwide,

Seriously concerned to forestall all forms of advertising, promotion, and sponsorship aimed at encouraging the use of cannabis products,

Recognizing that cooperative action is necessary to eliminate all forms of illicit trade in cannabis products, including smuggling, illicit manufacturing, and counterfeiting,

Acknowledging that cannabis control at all levels and particularly in developing countries and in countries with economies in transition requires substantial financial and technical resources,

Mindful of the social and economic difficulties that cannabis control programmes may engender in the medium and long term in some developing countries and countries with economies in transition, and recognizing their need for technical and financial assistance in the context of nationally developed strategies for sustainable development,

Conscious of the valuable work being conducted by many States on cannabis control and commending the leadership of the Commission on Narcotic

Drugs, the UN Office on Drugs and Crime, and the WHO as well as the efforts of other organizations and bodies of the United Nations system and other international and regional intergovernmental organizations on drug control,

Emphasizing the special contribution of nongovernmental organizations and other members of civil society, including health professional bodies, women's, youth, environmental, and consumer groups, and academic and health care institutions, to cannabis control efforts nationally and internationally and the vital importance of their participation in national and international cannabis control efforts,

Recognizing the need to be alert to any efforts by producers or distributors of cannabis products to undermine or subvert control efforts, and the need to be informed of activities of those involved in the cannabis market that have a negative impact on cannabis control efforts,

Recalling Article 12 of the International Covenant on Economic, Social and Cultural Rights, adopted by the United Nations General Assembly on 16 December 1966, which states that it is the right of everyone to the enjoyment of the highest attainable standard of physical and mental health,

Recalling also the preamble to the Constitution of the WHO, which states that the enjoyment of the highest attainable standard of health is one of the fundamental rights of every human being without distinction of race, religion, political belief, economic, or social condition,

Determined to promote measures of cannabis control based on current and relevant scientific, technical, and economic considerations,

Have agreed, as follows:

Part I: Introduction

Article 1

Use of terms

For the purposes of this Convention:

(a) 'illicit trade' means any practice or conduct prohibited by law and which relates to production, shipment, receipt, possession, distribution, sale, or purchase including any practice or conduct intended to facilitate such activity;

(b) 'regional economic integration organization' means an organization that is composed of several sovereign states, and to which its Member States have transferred competence over a range of matters, including the authority to make decisions binding on its Member States in respect of those matters;[19]

(c) 'cannabis advertising and promotion' means any form of commercial communication, recommendation, or action with the aim, effect or likely effect of promoting a psychoactive cannabis product or cannabis use either directly or indirectly;

(d) 'cannabis control' means a range of supply, demand, and harm reduction strategies that aim to improve the health of a population by eliminating or reducing their consumption of cannabis products and exposure to cannabis smoke;

(e) 'cannabis industry' means cannabis manufacturers, wholesale distributors, and importers of cannabis products;

(f) 'cannabis products' means products entirely or partly made of any part of the cannabis plant as raw material which are manufactured or sold to be used for smoking, sucking, chewing , snuffing, or other human consumption;

(g) 'cannabis sponsorship' means any form of contribution to any event, activity, or individual with the aim, effect, or likely effect of promoting a cannabis product or cannabis use either directly or indirectly;

(h) 'cannabis for personal use' means a limited amount of cannabis or cannabis products, with maximum amounts set by legislation, which is cultivated or kept for personal or shared use without any remuneration or other consideration;

Article 2

Relationship between this Convention and other agreements and legal instruments

1 In order to better protect human health, Parties may implement measures beyond those required by this Convention and its protocols, and nothing in these instruments shall prevent a Party from imposing stricter requirements that are consistent with their provisions and are in accordance with international law.

2 The provisions of the Convention and its protocols shall in no way affect the right of Parties to enter into bilateral or multilateral agreements, including regional or subregional agreements, on issues relevant or

---

[19] Where appropriate, national will refer equally to regional economic integration organizations.

additional to the Convention and its protocols, provided that such agreements are compatible with their obligations under the Convention and its protocols. The Parties concerned shall communicate such agreements to the Conference of the Parties through the Secretariat.

Part II: Objective, guiding principles and general obligations

Article 3

Objective

1 The objective of this Convention and its protocols is to provide a framework for cannabis control measures to be implemented by the Parties at the national, regional, and international levels, thereby:

   (a) Supporting States which legally provide for nonmedical sale or use to structure and control the market for cannabis products so as to minimize social and health harm from use;

   (b) Supporting the cannabis control policies of States where nonmedical cannabis sale or use is prohibited.

2 This Convention shall not apply to the cultivation of the cannabis plant exclusively for industrial purposes (fibre and seed) or horticultural purposes.

3 The Parties shall adopt such measures as may be necessary to prevent illicit traffic in the leaves of the cannabis plant.

Article 4

Guiding principles

To achieve the objective of this Convention and its protocols and to implement its provisions, the Parties shall be guided, *inter alia*, by the principles set out below:

1 Every person should be informed of the risk of health consequences and potential addictive nature of cannabis consumption, especially of long-term frequent use.

2 Strong political commitment is necessary to develop and support, at the national, regional, and international levels, comprehensive multisectoral measures and coordinated responses.

3 International cooperation, particularly transfer of technology, knowledge and financial assistance and provision of related expertise, to establish and

implement effective cannabis control programmes, taking into consideration local culture, as well as social, economic, political, and legal factors, is an important part of the Convention.

4 Comprehensive multisectoral measures and responses at the national, regional, and international levels are essential so as to prevent, in accordance with public health principles, the incidence of diseases, premature disability, and mortality due to cannabis consumption.

5 The participation of civil society is essential in achieving the objective of the Convention and its protocols.

Article 5

General obligations

1 Each Party shall develop, implement, periodically update and review comprehensive multisectoral national cannabis control strategies, plans and programmes in accordance with this Convention and the protocols to which it is a Party.

2 Towards this end, each Party shall, in accordance with its capabilities:

   (a) establish or reinforce and finance a national coordinating mechanism or focal points for cannabis control; and

   (b) adopt and implement effective legislative, executive, administrative, and/or other measures and cooperate, as appropriate, with other Parties in developing appropriate policies for cannabis control.

3 In setting and implementing their public health policies with respect to cannabis control, Parties shall act to protect these policies from commercial and other vested economic interests, including those of the cannabis industry.

4 The Parties shall cooperate in the formulation of proposed measures, procedures, and guidelines for the implementation of the Convention and the protocols to which they are Parties.

5 The Parties shall cooperate, as appropriate, with competent international and regional intergovernmental organizations and other bodies to achieve the objectives of the Convention and the protocols to which they are Parties.

6 The Parties shall, within means and resources at their disposal, cooperate to raise financial resources for effective implementation of the Convention through bilateral and multilateral funding mechanisms.

Part III: Measures relating to the reduction of demand for cannabis

Article 6

Price and tax measures to reduce the demand for cannabis

1 The Parties recognize that price and tax measures are an effective and important means of controlling cannabis consumption by various segments of the population, in particular young persons.

2 Without prejudice to the sovereign right of the Parties to determine and establish their taxation policies, each Party should take account of its national health objectives concerning cannabis control and adopt or maintain, as appropriate, measures which may include:

   (a) implementing tax policies and, where appropriate, price policies, on cannabis products so as to contribute to the health objectives aimed at minimizing harmful patterns of cannabis consumption; and

   (b) prohibiting or restricting, as appropriate, sales to and/or importations by international travellers of tax- and duty-free cannabis products.

3 The Parties shall provide rates of taxation for cannabis products and trends in cannabis consumption in their periodic reports to the Conference of the Parties, in accordance with Article 21.

Article 7

Non-price measures to reduce the demand for cannabis

The Parties recognize that comprehensive non-price measures are an effective and important means of reducing cannabis consumption. Each Party shall adopt and implement effective legislative, executive, administrative, or other measures necessary to implement its obligations pursuant to Articles 8–13 and shall cooperate, as appropriate, with each other directly or through competent international bodies with a view to their implementation. The Conference of the Parties shall propose appropriate guidelines for the implementation of the provisions of these Articles.

Article 8

Regulation of the production and sale of cannabis

1 If a Party permits the cultivation of the cannabis plant for the production of cannabis other than for personal use, it shall maintain one or more

government agencies (hereinafter referred to in this article as the Agency) to carry out the functions required by this article.

2 A Party may choose to allow cultivation and possession of cannabis or cannabis products for personal use, within upper limits on amounts which are set by legislation. Such cannabis for personal use may be exempted from sections 3 and 4 below.

3 The Agency shall designate the areas in which, and the plots of land on which, cultivation of cannabis for use in cannabis products shall be permitted. Only cultivators licensed by the Agency shall be authorized to engage in such cultivation. Each license shall specify the extent of the land or the premises on which the cultivation is permitted.

4 All cultivators are required to deliver their total crops to the Agency or to one or more licensed wholesalers or manufacturers. The cannabis which is cultivated must be put in the physical possession of the Agency, wholesaler or manufacturer no later than four months after the end of the harvest.

5 The Parties shall require that each wholesaler and manufacturer of cannabis and cannabis products be under licence, except where the wholesaler or manufacturer is a State enterprise. The Parties shall: (a) Control all persons and enterprises carrying on or engaged in the wholesaling or manufacture of cannabis or cannabis products; (b) Control under licence the establishments and premises in which such wholesaling or manufacture may take place; (c) Require that licensed wholesalers and manufacturers obtain periodical permits specifying the kinds and amounts of products they shall be entitle to manufacture or handle, and that they meet specified standards of quality control.

6 The Parties shall require that trade in, distribution of, and places for use of cannabis and cannabis products be under licence except where such trade or distribution is carried out by a State enterprise. The Parties shall: (a) Control all persons and enterprises carrying on or engaged in the trade or distribution of cannabis or cannabis products; (b) Control under licence the establishments and premises in which such trade, distribution, or provision may take place; (c) Require that licensed traders, distributors, and keepers of premises for use obtain periodical permits specifying the conditions of trade and distribution; (d) Specify hours and days when places for sale or use may be open for business; (e) Provide means for effective enforcement of cannabis controls, with provision for licenses to be suspended or revoked for non-compliance.

Article 9

Sales to and by minors

1 Each Party shall adopt and implement effective legislative, executive, administrative, or other measures at the appropriate government level to prohibit the sales of cannabis products to persons under the age set by domestic law, national law, or eighteen. These measures may include:

   (a) requiring that all sellers of cannabis products place a clear and prominent indicator inside their point of sale about the prohibition of cannabis sales to minors and, in case of doubt, request that each cannabis purchaser provide appropriate evidence of having reached full legal age;

   (b) banning the sale of cannabis products in any manner by which they are directly accessible, such as store shelves; and

   (c) prohibiting the manufacture and sale of sweets, snacks, toys, or any other objects in the form of cannabis products which appeal to minors.

2 Each Party shall prohibit or promote the prohibition of the distribution of free cannabis products to the public and especially minors.

3 The Parties recognize that in order to increase their effectiveness, measures to prevent cannabis product sales to minors should, where appropriate, be implemented in conjunction with other provisions contained in this Convention.

4 Each party shall prohibit the introduction or use of cannabis vending machines within its jurisdiction.

5 Each Party shall adopt and implement effective legislative, executive, administrative, or other measures, including penalties against sellers and distributors, in order to ensure compliance with the obligations contained in paragraphs 1–4 of this Article.

6 Each Party should, as appropriate, adopt and implement effective legislative, executive, administrative, or other measures to prohibit the sales of cannabis products by persons under the age set by domestic law, national law, or eighteen.

Article 10

Regulation of the contents of and disclosures concerning cannabis products

1 The Conference of the Parties, in consultation with competent international bodies, shall propose guidelines for testing and measuring the contents

and emissions of cannabis products, and for the regulation of these contents and emissions. Each Party shall, where approved by competent national authorities, adopt and implement effective legislative, executive, and administrative or other measures for such testing and measuring, and for such regulation.

2 Each Party shall, in accordance with its national law, adopt and implement effective legislative, executive, administrative, or other measures requiring manufacturers and importers of cannabis products to disclose to governmental authorities information about the contents and emissions of cannabis products. Each Party shall further adopt and implement effective measures for public disclosure of information about the toxic constituents of the cannabis products and the emissions that they may produce.

Article 11

Packaging and labelling of cannabis products

1 Each Party shall adopt and implement, in accordance with its national law, effective measures to ensure that:

(a) cannabis product packaging and labelling do not promote a cannabis product by any means. Further, any cannabis product packaging and labelling shall not provide information that is false, misleading, deceptive or likely to create an erroneous impression about its characteristics, health effects, hazards, or emission.; and

(b) each unit packet and package of cannabis products and any outside packaging and labelling of such products also carry health warnings describing the harmful effects of cannabis use, and may include other appropriate messages, including information on laws which apply and treatment referral information . These warnings and messages:

　(i) shall be approved by the competent national authority,

　(ii) shall be rotating,

　(iii) shall be large, clear, visible, and legible,

　(iv) should be 50% or more of the principal display areas but shall be no less than 30% of the principal display areas,

　(v) may be in the form of or include pictures or pictograms.

2 Each unit packet and package of cannabis products and any outside packaging and labelling of such products shall, in addition to the warnings specified in paragraph 1(b) of this Article, contain information on relevant constituents and emissions of cannabis products as defined by national authorities.

3 Each Party shall require that the warnings and other textual information specified in paragraphs 1(b) and paragraph 2 of this Article will appear on each unit packet and package of cannabis products and any outside packaging and labelling of such products in its principal language or languages.

4 For the purposes of this Article, the term 'outside packaging and labelling' in relation to cannabis products applies to any packaging and labelling used in the retail sale of the product.

Article 12

Education, communication, training, and public awareness

Each Party shall promote and strengthen public awareness of cannabis control issues, using all available communication tools, as appropriate. Towards this end, each Party shall adopt and implement effective legislative, executive, administrative, or other measures to promote:

(a) broad access to effective and comprehensive educational and public awareness programmes on the health risks including the addictive characteristics of cannabis consumption;

(b) public awareness about the health risks of cannabis consumption smoke, and about the benefits of the cessation of cannabis use and cannabis-free lifestyles as specified in Article 14.2;

(c) effective and appropriate training or sensitization and awareness programmes on cannabis control addressed to persons such as health workers, community workers, social workers, media professionals, educators, decision-makers, administrators, and other concerned persons;

(d) awareness and participation of public and private agencies and non-governmental organizations in developing and implementing inter-sectoral programmes and strategies for cannabis control; and

(e) public awareness of and access to information regarding adverse health and other consequences of cannabis production and consumption.

Article 13

Cannabis advertising, promotion, and sponsorship

1 Parties recognize that a comprehensive ban on advertising, promotion, and sponsorship will tend to reduce the consumption of cannabis products.

2 Each Party shall, in accordance with its constitution or constitutional principles, undertake a comprehensive ban of all cannabis advertising, promotion, and sponsorship. This shall include, subject to the legal environment and technical means available to that Party, a comprehensive ban on cross-border advertising, promotion, and sponsorship originating from its territory. In this respect, within the period of five years after entry into force of this Convention for that Party, each Party shall undertake appropriate legislative, executive, administrative, and/or other measures and report accordingly in conformity with Article 21.

3 A Party that is not in a position to undertake a comprehensive ban due to its constitution or constitutional principles shall apply restrictions on all cannabis advertising, promotion, and sponsorship. This shall include, subject to the legal environment and technical means available to that Party, restrictions or a comprehensive ban on advertising, promotion, and sponsorship originating from its territory with cross-border effects. In this respect, each Party shall undertake appropriate legislative, executive, administrative, and/or other measures and report accordingly in conformity with Article 21.

4 As a minimum, and in accordance with its constitution or constitutional principles, each Party shall:

    (a) prohibit all forms of cannabis advertising, promotion, and sponsorship that promote a cannabis product by any means that are false, misleading or deceptive or likely to create an erroneous impression about its characteristics, health effects, hazards, or emissions;

    (b) require that health or other appropriate warnings or messages accompany all cannabis advertising and, as appropriate, promotion and sponsorship;

    (c) restrict the use of direct or indirect incentives that encourage the purchase of cannabis products by the public;

    (d) require, if it does not have a comprehensive ban, the disclosure to relevant governmental authorities of expenditures by the cannabis industry on advertising, promotion, and sponsorship not yet prohibited. The Party should make those figures available, subject to national law, to the public and to the Conference of the Parties, pursuant to Article 21;

    (e) undertake a comprehensive ban or, in the case of a Party that is not in a position to undertake a comprehensive ban due to its constitution or constitutional principles, restrict cannabis advertising, promotion, and sponsorship on radio, television, print media and, as appropriate, other media, such as the internet, within a period of five years; and

(f) prohibit, or in the case of a Party that is not in a position to prohibit due to its constitution or constitutional principles restrict, cannabis industry sponsorship of international events, activities and/or participants therein.

5 Parties are encouraged to implement measures beyond the obligations set out in paragraph 4.

6 Parties shall cooperate in the development of technologies and other means necessary to facilitate the elimination of cross-border advertising.

7 Parties which have a ban on certain forms of cannabis advertising, promotion, and sponsorship have the sovereign right to ban those forms of cross-border cannabis advertising, promotion, and sponsorship entering their territory and to impose equal penalties as those applicable to domestic advertising, promotion, and sponsorship originating from their territory in accordance with their national law. This paragraph does not endorse or approve of any particular penalty.

8 Parties shall consider the elaboration of a protocol setting out appropriate measures that require international collaboration for a comprehensive ban on cross-border advertising, promotion, and sponsorship.

Article 14

Demand reduction measures concerning cannabis dependence and cessation or limitation of use

1 Each Party shall develop and disseminate appropriate, comprehensive, and integrated guidelines based on scientific evidence and best practices, taking into account national circumstances and priorities, and shall take effective measures to promote cessation or limitation of cannabis use and adequate treatment for cannabis dependence.

2 Towards this end, each Party shall endeavour to:

(a) design and implement effective programmes aimed at promoting the cessation or limitation of cannabis use, in such locations as educational institutions, health care facilities, workplaces, and sporting environments;

(b) include diagnosis and treatment of cannabis dependence and counselling services on cessation or limitation of cannabis use in national health and education programmes, plans, and strategies, with the participation of health workers, community workers, and social workers as appropriate;

(c) establish in health care facilities and rehabilitation centres programmes for diagnosing, counselling, preventing, and treating cannabis dependence; and

(d) collaborate with other Parties to facilitate accessibility and affordability for treatment of cannabis dependence including pharmaceutical products pursuant to Article 22. Such products and their constituents may include medicines, products used to administer medicines and diagnostics when appropriate.

Part IV: Measures relating to controlling legal trade and suppressing illegal trade in cannabis

Article 15

Illicit trade in cannabis products

1 The Parties recognize that the elimination of all forms of illicit trade in cannabis products, including smuggling, illicit manufacturing and counterfeiting, and the development and implementation of related national law, in addition to subregional, regional, and global agreements, are essential components of cannabis control.

2 Each Party shall adopt and implement effective legislative, executive, administrative, or other measures to ensure that all unit packets and packages of cannabis products and any outside packaging of such products are marked to assist Parties in determining the origin of cannabis products, and in accordance with national law and relevant bilateral or multilateral agreements, assist Parties in determining the point of diversion and monitor, document, and control the movement of cannabis products and their legal status. In addition, each Party shall:

(a) require that unit packets and packages of cannabis products for retail and wholesale use that are sold on its domestic market carry the statement: *'Sales only allowed in (insert name of the country, subnational, regional or federal unit)'* or carry any other effective marking indicating the final destination or which would assist authorities in determining whether the product is legally for sale on the domestic market; and

(b) develop a practical tracking and tracing regime in compliance with Article 16 that would further secure the distribution system and assist in the investigation of illicit trade.

3 Each Party shall require that the packaging information or marking specified in paragraph 2 of this Article shall be presented in legible form and/or appear in its principal language or languages.

4 With a view to eliminating illicit trade in cannabis products, each Party shall:

    (a) monitor and collect data on cross-border trade in cannabis products, including illicit trade, and exchange information among customs, tax, and other authorities, as appropriate, and in accordance with national law and relevant applicable bilateral or multilateral agreements;

    (b) enact or strengthen legislation, with appropriate penalties and remedies, against illicit trade in cannabis products, including counterfeit and contraband cannabis cigarettes;

    (c) take appropriate steps to ensure that all confiscated manufacturing equipment, counterfeit and contraband cannabis and cannabis products are destroyed, using environmentally friendly methods where feasible, or disposed of in accordance with national law;

    (d) adopt and implement measures to monitor, document, and control the storage and distribution of cannabis and cannabis products held or moving under suspension of taxes or duties within its jurisdiction; and

    (e) adopt measures as appropriate to enable the confiscation of proceeds derived from the illicit trade in cannabis products.

5 Information collected pursuant to subparagraphs 4(a) and 4(d) of this Article shall, as appropriate, be provided in aggregate form by the Parties in their periodic reports to the Conference of the Parties, in accordance with Article 21.

6 The Parties shall, as appropriate and in accordance with national law, promote cooperation between national agencies, as well as relevant regional and international intergovernmental organizations as it relates to investigations, prosecutions, and proceedings, with a view to eliminating illicit trade in cannabis products. Special emphasis shall be placed on cooperation at regional and subregional levels to combat illicit trade of cannabis products.

7 Each Party shall endeavour to adopt and implement further measures including licensing, where appropriate, to control or regulate the production and distribution of cannabis products in order to prevent illicit trade.

Article 16

Provisions relating to international trade

1 The Parties shall not knowingly permit the export of cannabis or cannabis products to any country or territory except in accordance with the laws and regulations of that country or territory.

2 The Parties shall exercise in free ports and zones the same supervision and control as in other parts of their territories, provided, however, that they may apply more drastic measures.

3 The Parties shall:

(a) Control under licence the import and export of cannabis and cannabis products except where such import or export is carried out by a State enterprise.

(b) Control all persons and enterprises carrying on or engaged in such import or export.

4 (a) Every Party permitting the import or export of cannabis or cannabis products shall require a separate import or export authorization to be obtained for each import or export. The authorization may allow an importation or exportation in more than one consignment.

(b) Such authorization shall state the form of the cannabis product, the quantity to be imported or exported, and the name and address of the importer and exporter, and shall specify the period in which the importation or exportation must be effected.

(c) The export authorization shall also state the number and date of the import certificate (paragraph 5) and the authority by whom it has been issued.

5 Before issuing an export authorization the Parties shall require an import certificate, issued by the competent authorities of the importing country or territory and certifying that the importation referred to therein is approved, and such certificate shall be produced by the person or establishment applying for the export authorization.

6 A copy of the export authorization shall accompany each consignment and the Government issuing the export authorization shall send a copy to the Government of the importing country or territory.

7 (a) The Government of the importing country or territory, when the importation has been effected or when the period fixed for the importation has expired, shall return the export authorization with an endorsement to that effect, to the Government of the exporting country or territory.

(b) The endorsement shall specify the amount actually imported.

(c) If a lesser quantity than that specified in the export authorization is actually exported, the quantity actually exported shall be stated by the competent authorities on the export authorization and on any official copy thereof.

8 Exports of consignments to a post office box, or to a bank to the account of a party other than the party named in the export authorization, shall be prohibited.

9 Exports of consignments to a bonded warehouse are prohibited unless the Government of the importing country certifies on the import certificate, produced by the person or establishment applying for the export authorization, that it has approved the importation for the purpose of being placed in a bonded warehouse. In such case the export authorization shall specify that the consignment is exported for such a purpose. Each withdrawal from the bonded warehouse shall require a permit from the authorities having jurisdiction over the warehouse and, in the case of a foreign destination, shall be treated as if it were a new export within the meaning of the Convention.

10 Consignments of drugs entering or leaving the territory of a Party not accompanied by an export authorization shall be detained by the competent authorities.

11 A party shall not permit any cannabis or cannabis products consigned to another country to pass through its territory, whether or not the consignment is removed from the conveyance in which it is carried, unless a copy of the export authorization for such a consignment is produced to the competent authorities of such Party.

12 The competent authorities of any country or territory through which a consignment of drugs is permitted to pass shall take all due measures to prevent the diversion of the consignment to a destination other than that named in the accompanying copy of the export authorization unless the Government of that country or territory through which the consignment is passing authorizes the diversion. The Government of the country or territory of transit shall treat any requested diversion as if the diversion were an export from the country or territory of transit to the country or territory of new destination. If the diversion is authorized, the provisions of paragraph 7(a) and (b) shall also apply between the country or territory of transit and the country or territory which originally exported the consignment.

13 No consignment of cannabis or cannabis products while in transit, or while being stored in a bonded warehouse, may be subjected to any process which would change its nature. The packing may not be altered without the permission of the competent authorities.

14 The provisions of paragraphs 11 to 13 relating to the passage of cannabis or cannabis products through the territory of a Party do not apply where the consignment in question is transported by aircraft which does not land in the country or territory of transit. If the aircraft lands in any such country or territory, those provisions shall be applied so far as circumstances require.

15 Except as provided in paragraph 16, the provisions of this article are without prejudice to the provisions of any international agreements which limit the control which may be exercised by any of the Parties over drugs in transit.

16 In view of the health and social harms which can result from the use of cannabis or cannabis products, this convention takes precedence over any international agreement or treaty which provides for free movement or equitable treatment of goods or services in trade or commerce.

Article 17

Provision of support for economically viable alternative activities

Parties shall, in cooperation with each other and with competent international and regional intergovernmental organizations, promote, as appropriate, economically viable alternatives for cannabis workers, growers and, as the case may be, individual sellers.

Part V: Protection of the environment

Article 18

Protection of the environment and the health of persons

In carrying out their obligations under this Convention, the Parties agree to have due regard to the protection of the environment and the health of persons in relation to the environment in respect of cannabis cultivation and manufacture within their respective territories.

Part VI: Questions related to liability

Article 19

Liability

1 For the purpose of cannabis control, the Parties shall consider taking legislative action or promoting their existing laws, where necessary, to deal with criminal and civil liability, including compensation where appropriate.

2 Parties shall cooperate with each other in exchanging information through the Conference of the Parties in accordance with Article 21 including:

   (a) information on the health effects of the consumption of cannabis products in accordance with Article 20.3(a); and

   (b) information on legislation and regulations in force as well as pertinent jurisprudence.

3 The Parties shall, as appropriate and mutually agreed, within the limits of national legislation, policies, legal practices, and applicable existing treaty arrangements, afford one another assistance in legal proceedings relating to civil and criminal liability consistent with this Convention.

4 The Convention shall in no way affect or limit any rights of access of the Parties to each other's courts where such rights exist.

5 The Conference of the Parties may consider, if possible, at an early stage, taking account of the work being done in relevant international fora, issues related to liability including appropriate international approaches to these issues and appropriate means to support, upon request, the Parties in their legislative and other activities in accordance with this Article.

Part VII: Scientific and technical cooperation and communication of information

Article 20

Research, surveillance, and exchange of information

1 The Parties undertake to develop and promote national research and to coordinate research programmes at the regional and international levels in the field of cannabis control. Towards this end, each Party shall:

(a) initiate and cooperate in, directly or through competent international and regional intergovernmental organizations and other bodies, the conduct of research and scientific assessments, and in so doing promote and encourage research that addresses the determinants and consequences of cannabis consumption as well as research for identification of alternative crops; and

(b) promote and strengthen, with the support of competent international and regional intergovernmental organizations and other bodies, training and support for all those engaged in cannabis control activities, including research, implementation, and evaluation.

2 The Parties shall establish, as appropriate, programmes for national, regional, and global surveillance of the magnitude, patterns, determinants, and consequences of cannabis consumption. Towards this end, the Parties should integrate cannabis surveillance programmes into national, regional, and global health surveillance programmes so that data are comparable and can be analysed at the regional and international levels, as appropriate.

3 Parties recognize the importance of financial and technical assistance from international and regional intergovernmental organizations and other bodies. Each Party shall endeavour to:

(a) establish progressively a national system for the epidemiological surveillance of cannabis consumption and related social, economic, and health indicators;

(b) cooperate with competent international and regional intergovernmental organizations and other bodies, including governmental and nongovernmental agencies, in regional and global cannabis surveillance and exchange of information on the indicators specified in paragraph 3(a) of this Article; and

(c) cooperate with the WHO in the development of general guidelines or procedures for defining the collection, analysis and dissemination of cannabis-related surveillance data.

4 The Parties shall, subject to national law, promote and facilitate the exchange of publicly available scientific, technical, socioeconomic, commercial, and legal information, as well as information regarding practices of the cannabis industry and the cultivation of cannabis, which is relevant to this Convention, and in so doing shall take into account and address the special needs of developing country Parties and Parties with economies in transition. Each Party shall endeavour to:

(a) progressively establish and maintain an updated database of laws and regulations on cannabis control and, as appropriate, information about their enforcement, as well as pertinent jurisprudence, and cooperate in the development of programmes for regional and global cannabis control;

(b) progressively establish and maintain updated data from national surveillance programmes in accordance with paragraph 3(a) of this Article; and

(c) cooperate with competent international organizations to progressively establish and maintain a global system to regularly collect and disseminate information on cannabis production, manufacture, and the activities of the cannabis industry which have an impact on the Convention or national cannabis control activities.

5 Parties should cooperate in regional and international intergovernmental organizations and financial and development institutions of which they are members, to promote and encourage provision of technical and financial resources to the Secretariat to assist developing country Parties and

Parties with economies in transition to meet their commitments on research, surveillance, and exchange of information.

Article 21

Reporting and exchange of information

1 Each Party shall submit to the Conference of the Parties, through the Secretariat, periodic reports on its implementation of this Convention, which should include the following:

  (a) information on legislative, executive, administrative, or other measures taken to implement the Convention;

  (b) information, as appropriate, on any constraints or barriers encountered in its implementation of the Convention, and on the measures taken to overcome these barriers;

  (c) information, as appropriate, on financial and technical assistance provided or received for cannabis control activities;

  (d) information on surveillance and research as specified in Article 20; and

  (e) information specified in Articles 6.3, 13.2, 13.3, 13.4(d), 15.5, and 19.2.

2 The frequency and format of such reports by all Parties shall be determined by the Conference of the Parties. Each Party shall make its initial report within two years of the entry into force of the Convention for that Party.

3 The Conference of the Parties, pursuant to Articles 22 and 26, shall consider arrangements to assist developing country Parties and Parties with economies in transition, at their request, in meeting their obligations under this Article.

4 The reporting and exchange of information under the Convention shall be subject to national law regarding confidentiality and privacy. The Parties shall protect, as mutually agreed, any confidential information that is exchanged.

Article 22

Cooperation in the scientific, technical, and legal fields and provision of related expertise

1 The Parties shall cooperate directly or through competent international bodies to strengthen their capacity to fulfil the obligations arising from this Convention, taking into account the needs of developing country Parties and Parties with economies in transition. Such cooperation shall promote the transfer of technical, scientific, and legal expertise and technology, as

mutually agreed, to establish and strengthen national cannabis control strategies, plans, and programmes aiming at, *inter alia*:

(a) facilitation of the development, transfer, and acquisition of technology, knowledge, skills, capacity, and expertise related to cannabis control;

(b) provision of technical, scientific, legal, and other expertise to establish and strengthen national cannabis control strategies, plans, and programmes, aiming at implementation of the Convention through, *inter alia*:

 (i) assisting, upon request, in the development of a strong legislative foundation as well as technical programmes, including those on prevention of initiation, and promotion of cessation or limitation of use;

 (ii) assisting, as appropriate, cannabis workers in the development of appropriate economically and legally viable alternative livelihoods in an economically viable manner; and

 (iii) assisting, as appropriate, cannabis growers in shifting agricultural production to alternative crops in an economically viable manner;

(c) support for appropriate training or sensitization programmes for appropriate personnel in accordance with Article 12;

(d) provision, as appropriate, of the necessary material, equipment, and supplies, as well as logistical support, for cannabis control strategies, plans, and programmes;

(e) identification of methods for cannabis control, including comprehensive treatment of cannabis dependence; and

(f) promotion, as appropriate, of research to increase the affordability of comprehensive treatment of cannabis dependence.

2 The Conference of the Parties shall promote and facilitate transfer of technical, scientific, and legal expertise and technology with the financial support secured in accordance with Article 26.

Part VIII: Institutional arrangements and financial resources

Article 23

Conference of the Parties

1 A Conference of the Parties is hereby established. The first session of the Conference shall be convened by the WHO not later than one year after

the entry into force of this Convention. The Conference will determine the venue and timing of subsequent regular sessions at its first session.

2 Extraordinary sessions of the Conference of the Parties shall be held at such other times as may be deemed necessary by the Conference, or at the written request of any Party, provided that, within six months of the request being communicated to them by the Secretariat of the Convention, it is supported by at least one-third of the Parties.

3 The Conference of the Parties shall adopt by consensus its Rules of Procedure at its first session.

4 The Conference of the Parties shall by consensus adopt financial rules for itself as well as governing the funding of any subsidiary bodies it may establish as well as financial provisions governing the functioning of the Secretariat. At each ordinary session, it shall adopt a budget for the financial period until the next ordinary session.

5 The Conference of the Parties shall keep under regular review the implementation of the Convention and take the decisions necessary to promote its effective implementation and may adopt protocols, annexes, and amendments to the Convention, in accordance with Articles 28, 29, and 33. Towards this end, it shall:

(a) promote and facilitate the exchange of information pursuant to Articles 20 and 21;

(b) promote and guide the development and periodic refinement of comparable methodologies for research and the collection of data, in addition to those provided for in Article 20, relevant to the implementation of the Convention;

(c) promote, as appropriate, the development, implementation, and evaluation of strategies, plans, and programmes, as well as policies, legislation, and other measures;

(d) consider reports submitted by the Parties in accordance with Article 21 and adopt regular reports on the implementation of the Convention;

(e) promote and facilitate the mobilization of financial resources for the implementation of the Convention in accordance with Article 26;

(f) establish such subsidiary bodies as are necessary to achieve the objective of the Convention;

(g) request, where appropriate, the services and cooperation of, and information provided by, competent and relevant organizations and bodies of the United Nations system and other international and regional intergovernmental organizations and nongovernmental organizations and bodies as a means of strengthening the implementation of the Convention; and

(h) consider other action, as appropriate, for the achievement of the objective of the Convention in the light of experience gained in its implementation.

6 The Conference of the Parties shall establish the criteria for the participation of observers at its proceedings.

Article 24

Secretariat

1 The Conference of the Parties shall designate a permanent secretariat and make arrangements for its functioning. The Conference of the Parties shall endeavour to do so at its first session.

2 Until such time as a permanent secretariat is designated and established, secretariat functions under this Convention shall be provided by the WHO.

3 Secretariat functions shall be:

(a) to make arrangements for sessions of the Conference of the Parties and any subsidiary bodies and to provide them with services as required;

(b) to transmit reports received by it pursuant to the Convention;

(c) to provide support to the Parties, particularly developing country Parties and Parties with economies in transition, on request, in the compilation and communication of information required in accordance with the provisions of the Convention;

(d) to prepare reports on its activities under the Convention under the guidance of the Conference of the Parties and submit them to the Conference of the Parties;

(e) to ensure, under the guidance of the Conference of the Parties, the necessary coordination with the competent international and regional intergovernmental organizations and other bodies;

(f) to enter, under the guidance of the Conference of the Parties, into such administrative or contractual arrangements as may be required for the effective discharge of its functions; and

(g) to perform other secretariat functions specified by the Convention and by any of its protocols and such other functions as may be determined by the Conference of the Parties.

Article 25

Relations between the Conference of the Parties and intergovernmental organizations

In order to provide technical and financial cooperation for achieving the objective of this Convention, the Conference of the Parties may request the cooperation of competent international and regional intergovernmental organizations including financial and development institutions.

Article 26

Financial resources

1 The Parties recognize the important role that financial resources play in achieving the objective of this Convention.

2 Each Party shall provide financial support in respect of its national activities intended to achieve the objective of the Convention, in accordance with its national plans, priorities, and programmes.

3 Parties shall promote, as appropriate, the utilization of bilateral, regional, subregional, and other multilateral channels to provide funding for the development and strengthening of multisectoral comprehensive cannabis control programmes of developing country Parties and Parties with economies in transition. Accordingly, economically viable alternatives to cannabis production, including crop diversification should be addressed and supported in the context of nationally developed strategies of sustainable development.

4 Parties represented in relevant regional and international intergovernmental organizations, and financial and development institutions shall encourage these entities to provide financial assistance for developing country Parties and for Parties with economies in transition to assist them in meeting their obligations under the Convention, without limiting the rights of participation within these organizations.

5 The Parties agree that:

   (a) to assist Parties in meeting their obligations under the Convention, all relevant potential and existing resources, financial, technical, or otherwise, both public and private that are available for cannabis control activities, should be mobilized and utilized for the benefit of all Parties, especially developing countries and countries with economies in transition;

   (b) the Secretariat shall advise developing country Parties and Parties with economies in transition, upon request, on available sources of funding to facilitate the implementation of their obligations under the Convention;

(c) the Conference of the Parties in its first session shall review existing and potential sources and mechanisms of assistance based on a study conducted by the Secretariat and other relevant information, and consider their adequacy; and

(d) the results of this review shall be taken into account by the Conference of the Parties in determining the necessity to enhance existing mechanisms or to establish a voluntary global fund or other appropriate financial mechanisms to channel additional financial resources, as needed, to developing country Parties and Parties with economies in transition to assist them in meeting the objectives of the Convention.

Part IX: Settlement of disputes

Article 27

Settlement of disputes

1 In the event of a dispute between two or more Parties concerning the interpretation or application of this Convention, the Parties concerned shall seek through diplomatic channels a settlement of the dispute through negotiation or any other peaceful means of their own choice, including good offices, mediation, or conciliation. Failure to reach agreement by good offices, mediation, or conciliation shall not absolve parties to the dispute from the responsibility of continuing to seek to resolve it.

2 When ratifying, accepting, approving, formally confirming, or acceding to the Convention, or at any time thereafter, a State or regional economic integration organization may declare in writing to the Depositary that, for a dispute not resolved in accordance with paragraph 1 of this Article, it accepts, as compulsory, ad hoc arbitration in accordance with procedures to be adopted by consensus by the Conference of the Parties.

3 The provisions of this Article shall apply with respect to any protocol as between the parties to the protocol, unless otherwise provided therein.

Part X: Development of the convention

Article 28

Amendments to this Convention

1 Any Party may propose amendments to this Convention. Such amendments will be considered by the Conference of the Parties.

2 Amendments to the Convention shall be adopted by the Conference of the Parties. The text of any proposed amendment to the Convention shall be communicated to the Parties by the Secretariat at least six months before the session at which it is proposed for adoption. The Secretariat shall also communicate proposed amendments to the signatories of the Convention and, for information, to the Depositary.

3 The Parties shall make every effort to reach agreement by consensus on any proposed amendment to the Convention. If all efforts at consensus have been exhausted, and no agreement reached, the amendment shall as a last resort be adopted by a three-quarters majority vote of the Parties present and voting at the session. For purposes of this Article, Parties present and voting means Parties present and casting an affirmative or negative vote. Any adopted amendment shall be communicated by the Secretariat to the Depositary, who shall circulate it to all Parties for acceptance.

4 Instruments of acceptance in respect of an amendment shall be deposited with the Depositary. An amendment adopted in accordance with paragraph 3 of this Article shall enter into force for those Parties having accepted it on the ninetieth day after the date of receipt by the Depositary of an instrument of acceptance by at least two-thirds of the Parties to the Convention.

5 The amendment shall enter into force for any other Party on the ninetieth day after the date on which that Party deposits with the Depositary its instrument of acceptance of the said amendment.

Article 29

Adoption and amendment of annexes to this Convention

1 Annexes to this Convention and amendments thereto shall be proposed, adopted, and shall enter into force in accordance with the procedure set forth in Article 28.

2 Annexes to the Convention shall form an integral part thereof and, unless otherwise expressly provided, a reference to the Convention constitutes at the same time a reference to any annexes thereto.

3 Annexes shall be restricted to lists, forms, and any other descriptive material relating to procedural, scientific, technical, or administrative matters.

Part XI: Final provisions

Article 30

Reservations

No reservations may be made to this Convention.

Article 31

Withdrawal

1 At any time after two years from the date on which this Convention has entered into force for a Party, that Party may withdraw from the Convention by giving written notification to the Depositary.

2 Any such withdrawal shall take effect upon expiry of one year from the date of receipt by the Depositary of the notification of withdrawal, or on such later date as may be specified in the notification of withdrawal.

3 Any Party that withdraws from the Convention shall be considered as also having withdrawn from any protocol to which it is a Party.

Article 32

Right to vote

1 Each Party to this Convention shall have one vote, except as provided for in paragraph 2 of this Article.

2 Regional economic integration organizations, in matters within their competence, shall exercise their right to vote with a number of votes equal to the number of their Member States that are Parties to the Convention. Such an organization shall not exercise its right to vote if any of its Member States exercises its right, and vice versa.

Article 33

Protocols

1 Any Party may propose protocols. Such proposals will be considered by the Conference of the Parties.

2 The Conference of the Parties may adopt protocols to this Convention. In adopting these protocols every effort shall be made to reach consensus. If all efforts at consensus have been exhausted, and no agreement reached, the protocol shall as a last resort be adopted by a three-quarters majority vote of the Parties present and voting at the session. For the purposes of this Article, Parties present and voting means Parties present and casting an affirmative or negative vote.

3 The text of any proposed protocol shall be communicated to the Parties by the Secretariat at least six months before the session at which it is proposed for adoption.

4 Only Parties to the Convention may be parties to a protocol.

5 Any protocol to the Convention shall be binding only on the parties to the protocol in question. Only Parties to a protocol may take decisions on matters exclusively relating to the protocol in question.

6 The requirements for entry into force of any protocol shall be established by that instrument.

Article 34

Signature

This Convention shall be open for signature by all Members of the WHO and by any States that are not Members of the WHO but are members of the United Nations and by regional economic integration organizations at the WHO headquarters in Geneva from XX to YY, and thereafter at United Nations Headquarters in New York, from YY to ZZ.

Article 35

Ratification, acceptance, approval, formal confirmation, or accession

1 This Convention shall be subject to ratification, acceptance, approval, or accession by States and to formal confirmation or accession by regional economic integration organizations. It shall be open for accession from the day after the date on which the Convention is closed for signature. Instruments of ratification, acceptance, approval, formal confirmation, or accession shall be deposited with the Depositary.

2 Any regional economic integration organization which becomes a Party to the Convention without any of its Member States being a Party shall be bound by all the obligations under the Convention. In the case of those organizations, one or more of whose Member States is a Party to the Convention, the organization and its Member States shall decide on their respective responsibilities for the performance of their obligations under the Convention. In such cases, the organization and the Member States shall not be entitled to exercise rights under the Convention concurrently.

3 Regional economic integration organizations shall, in their instruments relating to formal confirmation or in their instruments of accession, declare the extent of their competence with respect to the matters governed by the Convention. These organizations shall also inform the Depositary, who shall in turn inform the Parties, of any substantial modification in the extent of their competence.

Article 36

Entry into force

1 This Convention shall enter into force on the ninetieth day following the date of deposit of the fortieth instrument of ratification, acceptance, approval, formal confirmation, or accession with the Depositary.

2 For each State that ratifies, accepts, or approves the Convention or accedes thereto after the conditions set out in paragraph 1 of this Article for entry into force have been fulfilled, the Convention shall enter into force on the ninetieth day following the date of deposit of its instrument of ratification, acceptance, approval or accession.

3 For each regional economic integration organization depositing an instrument of formal confirmation or an instrument of accession after the conditions set out in paragraph 1 of this Article for entry into force have been fulfilled, the Convention shall enter into force on the ninetieth day following the date of its depositing of the instrument of formal confirmation or of accession.

4 For the purposes of this Article, any instrument deposited by a regional economic integration organization shall not be counted as additional to those deposited by States Members of the organization.

Article 37

Depositary

The Secretary-General of the United Nations shall be the Depositary of this Convention and amendments thereto and of protocols and annexes adopted in accordance with Articles 28, 29, and 33.

Article 38

Authentic texts

The original of this Convention, of which the Arabic, Chinese, English, French, Russian, and Spanish texts are equally authentic, shall be deposited with the Secretary-General of the United Nations.

IN WITNESS WHEREOF the undersigned, being duly authorized to that effect, have signed this Convention.

DONE at [PLACE] this [DATE].

References

Abel, D. (2008). Officials look for guidelines on marijuana initiative. *Boston Globe*, 6 November, p. B3. http://www.boston.com/news/local/massachusetts/ articles/2008/11/06/officials_look_for_guidelines_on_marijuana_initiative/

Abraham, M.D., Cohen, P.D.A. & Beukenhorst, D.J. (2001). Comparative cannabis use data. *British Journal of Psychiatry*, 179 (2): 175–7.

Adlaf, E.M., Begin, P. & Sawka, E. (eds.) (2005). *Canadian Addiction Survey (CAS): A national survey of Canadians' use of alcohol and other drugs: Prevalence of use and related harms: Detailed report.* Ottawa: Canadian Centre on Substance Abuse.

Advisory Council on the Misuse of Drugs (2008). *Cannabis: Classification and Public Health.* London: Home Office. Available at: http://drugs.homeoffice.gov.uk/.

Agrawal, A. & Lynskey, M.T. (2006). The genetic epidemiology of cannabis use, abuse and dependence. *Addiction*, 101: 801–12.

Agrawal, A., Lynskey, M.T., Bucholz, K.K., Martin, N.G., Madden, P.A. & Heath, A.C. (2007). Contrasting models of genetic co-morbidity for cannabis and other illicit drugs in adult Australian twins. *Psychological Medicine*, 37: 49–60.

AIHW (2006). *Closed Treatment Episodes: Client Profile by Principal Drug of Concern, AODTS-NMDS 2005–05.* Canberra: Australian Institute of Health and Welfare.

AIHW (2007). *Statistics on Drug Use in Australia, 2006.* Canberra: Australian Institute of Health and Welfare.

AIHW (2008). *2007 National Drug Strategy Household Survey: First Results.* Canberra: Australian Institute of Health and Welfare. Available at: http://www.aihw.gov.au/ publications/index.cfm/title/10579.

Ajdacic-Gross, V., Lauber, C., Warnke, I., Haker, H., Murray, R.M. & Rossler, W. (2007). Changing incidence of psychotic disorders among the young in Zurich. *Schizophrenia Research*, 95: 9–18.

Aldington, S., Williams, M., Nowitz, M., Weatherall, M., Pritchard, A., McNaughton, A., *et al.* (2007). Effects of cannabis on pulmonary structure, function and symptoms. *Thorax*, 62: 1058–63.

Aldington, S., Harwood, M., Cox, B., Weatherall, M., Beckert, L., Hansell, A., *et al.* (2008). Cannabis use and risk of lung cancer: A case-control study. *European Respiratory Journal*, 31: 280–6.

Aldrich, M.R. & Mikuriya, T. (1988). Savings in California law enforcement costs attributable to the Moscone Act of 1976 – a summary. *Journal of Drug Issues*, 20(1): 75–81.

Andenas, M. & Spivack, D. (2003). *The UN Drug Conventions Regime and Policy Reform.* London: British Institute of International and Comparative Law. http://www. senliscouncil.net/documents/BIICL_opinion.

Andréasson, S. & Allebeck, P. (1990). Cannabis and mortality among young men: A longitudinal study of Swedish conscripts. *Scandinavian Journal of Social Medicine*, 18: 9–15.

Andréasson, S., Engstrom, A., Allebeck, P. & Rydberg, U. (1987). Cannabis and schizophrenia: A longitudinal study of Swedish conscripts. *Lancet*, 2: 1483–6.

Angst, J. (1996). Comorbidity of mood disorders: A longitudinal prospective study. *British Journal of Psychiatry*, 168: 31–7.

Anonymous (2008). Europe: Czech lower house approves lower marijuana penalties. Available at: http://stopthedrugwar.org/chronicle/560/czech-repuiblic-marijuana-decriminalization

Anthony, J., Warner, L. & Kessler, R. (1994). Comparative epidemiology of dependence on tobacco, alcohol, controlled substances and inhalants: Basic findings from the National Comorbidity Study. *Experimental and Clinical Psychopharmacology*, 2: 244–68.

Anthony, J.C. (2006). The epidemiology of cannabis dependence. In: Roffman, R.A. & Stephens, R.S. (eds.), *Cannabis Dependence: Its Nature, Consequences and Treatment.* Cambridge, UK: Cambridge University Press, pp. 58–105.

Anthony, J.C. & Helzer, J.E. (1991). Syndromes of drug abuse and dependence. In: Robins, L.N. & Regier, D.A. (eds.), *Psychiatric Disorders in America: The Epidemiologic Catchment Area.* New York: Free Press, pp. 116–54.

Appel, J., Backes, G. & Robbins, J. (2004). California's Proposition 36: A success ripe for refinement and replication. *Criminology & Public Policy*, 3: 585–92.

Aronow, W. & Cassidy, J. (1974). Effect of marihuana and placebo marihuana smoking on angina pectoris. *New England Journal of Medicine*, 291: 65–7.

Aronow, W. & Cassidy, J. (1975). Effect of smoking marijuana and of a high nicotine cigarette on angina pectoris. *Clinical Pharmacology and Therapeutics*, 17: 549–54.

Arseneault, L., Cannon, M., Poulton, R., Murray, R., Caspi, A. & Moffitt, T. E. (2002). Cannabis use in adolescence and risk for adult psychosis: Longitudinal prospective study. *British Medical Journal*, 325: 1212–13.

Aryana, A. & Williams, M.A. (2007). Marijuana as a trigger of cardiovascular events: Speculation or scientific certainty? *International Journal of Cardiology*, 118: 141–4.

Asbridge, M., Poulin, C. & Donato, A. (2005). Motor vehicle collision risk and driving under the influence of cannabis: Evidence from adolescents in Atlantic Canada. *Accident Analysis and Prevention*, 37: 1025–34.

Ashworth, A. (2005). *Sentencing and Criminal Justice.* Cambridge: Cambridge University Press.

Atha, M., Blanchard, S. & Davis, S. (1999). *Regular Users II: UK Drugs Market Analysis, Purchasing Patterns, and Prices, 1997.* Independent Drug Monitoring Unit Publications, Wigan.

Aulinger, S. (1997). *Rechtsgleichheit und Rechtswirklichkeit bei der Strafverfolgung von Drogenkonsumenten.* Baden-Baden: Nomos.

Babor, T., Caetano, R., Casswell, S., Edwards, G., Giesbrecht, N., Graham, K. *et al.* (2003). *Alcohol: No ordinary commodity. Research and public policy.* Oxford and London: Oxford University Press.

Bachman, J.G., Wadsworth, K.N., O'Malley, P.M., Johnston, L.D. & Schulenberg, J. (1997). *Smoking, Drinking, and Drug Use in Young Adulthood: The Impacts of New Freedoms and New Responsibilities.* Mahwah, NJ: Lawrence Erlbaum.

Bachs, L. & Morland, H. (2001). Acute cardiovascular fatalities following cannabis use. *Forensic Science International*, 124: 200–03.

Baker, J. & Goh, D. (2004). *The Cannabis Cautioning Scheme Three Years On: An Implementation and Outcome Evaluation.* Sydney: New South Wales Bureau of Crime Statistics and Research.

Bammer, G., Hall, W. & Hamilton, M. (2002). Harm minimization in a prohibition context – Australia. *The Annals of the American Academy of Political and Social Science,* 582: 80–93.

Bates, M.N. & Blakely, T.A. (1999). Role of cannabis in motor vehicle crashes. *Epidemiologic Reviews,* 21: 222–32.

Bayley, D. (1994). *Police for the Future.* Oxford: Oxford University Press.

BBC News (2008). Swiss approve prescription heroin. *BBC News* website, November 30. http://news.bbc.co.uk/2/hi/europe/7757050.stm

BBC News (2009) Argentina rules on marijuana use. BBC News website, 26 August. http://news.bbc.co.uk/2/hi/americas/8221599.stm

Beautrais, A.L., Joyce, P.R. & Mulder, R.T. (1999). Cannabis abuse and serious suicide attempts. *Addiction,* 94: 1155–64.

Becker, G. & Murphy, K. (1988). A rational theory of addiction. *Journal of Political Economy,* 96: 675–700.

Beckett, K., Nyrop, K. & Pfingst, L. (2006). Race, drugs, and policing: Understanding disparities in drug delivery arrests. *Criminology,* 44: 105–37.

Bedard, M., Dubois, S. & Weaver, B. (2007). The impact of cannabis on driving. *Canadian Journal of Public Health,* 98: 6–11.

Begg, S., Vos, T., Barker, B., Stanley, L. & Lopez, A.D. (2007). *The Burden of Disease and Injury in Australia 2003.* Canberra: Australian Institute of Health and Welfare. Available at: http://www.aihw.gov.au/publications/index.cfm/title/10317.

Belenko, S. (2001). *Research on Drug Courts: A Critical Review 2001 Update.* New York: The National Center on Addiction and Substance Abuse (CASA) at Columbia University.

Bergmark, A. (2008). Treating cannabis use disorders: Perspectives and best practices. In: Rödner Sznitman, S., Olsson, B. & Room, R. (eds.), *A Cannabis Reader: Global Issues and Local Experiences,* Vol. 2, pp. 205–15. Lisbon: European Monitoring Center on Drugs and Drug Abuse.

Bewley-Taylor, D. (2004). Emerging policy contradictions between the UNODC 'universe' and the core values and mission of the UN. pp. 24–31. In: Senlis Council, *Global Drug Policy: Building a New Framework.* Paris: Senlis Council. http://www.senliscouncil.net/modules/publications/006_publication/documents/Taylor_paper

Bewley-Taylor, D. & Trace, M. (2006). *The International Narcotics Control Board: Watchdog or Guardian of the Conventions?* Beckley Foundation Report No. 7. Beckley, Oxon., UK: Beckley Foundation. http://www.beckleyfoundation.org/pdf/Report_07.pdf

Bilder, R., Volavka, J., Lachman, H. & Grace, A. (2004). The catechol-O-methyltransferase (COMT) polymorphism: Relations to the tonic-phasic dopamine hypothesis and neuropsychiatric phenotypes. *Neuropsychopharmacology,* 29: 1943–61.

Bloch, E. (1983). Effects of marijuana and cannabinoids on reproduction, endocrine function, development, and chromosomes. In: Fehr, K. & Kalant, H. (eds.), *Cannabis and Health Hazards.* Toronto: Addiction Research Foundation, pp. 355–432.

Block, R.I. & Ghoneim, M.M. (1993). Effects of chronic marijuana use on human cognition. *Psychopharmacology,* 110: 219–28.

Block, R.I., O'Leary, D.S., Ehrhardt, J.C., Augustinack, J.C., Ghoneim, M.M., Arndt, S., *et al.* (2000a). Effects of frequent marijuana use on brain tissue volume and composition. *Neuroreport*, 11: 491–6.

Block, R.I., O'Leary, D.S., Hichwa, R.D., Augustinack, J.C., Ponto, L.L.B., Ghoneim, M.M., *et al.* (2000b). Cerebellar hypoactivity in frequent marijuana users. *Neuroreport*, 11: 749–53.

Block, R.I., O'Leary, D.S., Hichwa, R.D., Augustinack, J.C., Ponto, L.L.B., Ghoneim, M.M., *et al.* (2002). Effects of frequent marijuana use on memory-related regional cerebral blood flow. *Pharmacology, Biochemistry and Behavior*, 72: 237–50.

Blows, S., Ivers, R.Q., Connor, J., Ameratunga, S., Woodward, M. & Norton, R. (2005). Marijuana use and car crash injury. *Addiction*, 100: 605–11.

Boekhout Van Solinge, T. (1999). Dutch drug policy in a European context. *Journal of Drug Issues*, 29: 511–28.

Bolla, K.I., Brown, K., Eldreth, D., Tate, K. & Cadet, J.L. (2002). Dose-related neurocognitive effects of marijuana use. *Neurology*, 59: 1337–43.

Bollinger, L. (2004). Drug law and policy in Germany and the European community: Recent developments. *Journal of Drug Issues*, 34: 491–509.

Bonnie, R. & Whitebread, C. (1974). *Marihuana Conviction – A History of Marihuana Prohibition in the United States*. Charlottesville: University Press of Virginia.

Borchers-Tempel, S. & Kolte, B. (2002). Cannabis consumption in Amsterdam, Bremen and San Francisco: A three-city comparison of long-term Cannabis consumption. *Journal of Drug Issues*, 32(2): 395–412.

Borges, G., Walters, E.E. & Kessler, R.C. (2000). Associations of substance use, abuse and dependence with subsequent suicidal behavior. *American Journal of Epidemiology*, 151: 781–9.

Bouchard, M. (2008). Towards a realistic method to estimate cannabis production in industrialized countries. *Contemporary Drug Problems*, 35: 291–320.

Bouchard, M., Alain, M. & Nguyen, H. (in press). Convenient labor: The prevalence and nature of youth involvement in the marijuana cultivation industry. *International Journal of Drug Policy*.

Boyd, N. (1986). *The Social Dimensions of Law*. Scarborough: Prentice-Hall Canada.

Boydell, J., van Os, J., Caspi, A., Kennedy, N., Giouroukou, E., Fearon, P., *et al.* (2006). Trends in cannabis use prior to first presentation with schizophrenia, in South-East London between 1965 and 1999. *Psychological Medicine*, 36: 1441–6.

Brady, P. (2004). Spanish stoner paradise. *Cannabis Culture Magazine* CC #47, 25 April. http://www.cannabisculture.com/articles/3257.html

Brook, J.S., Cohen, P. & Brook, D.W. (1998). Longitudinal study of co-occurring psychiatric disorders and substance use. *Journal of the American Academy of Child and Adolescent Psychiatry*, 37: 322–30.

Brooks, A., Stothard, C., Moss, J., Christie, P. & Ali, R. (1999). *Costs Associated with the Operation of the Cannabis Expiation Notice Scheme in South Australia*. Adelaide: Drug and Alcohol Services Council.

Brown, T.T. & Dobs, A.S. (2002). Endocrine effects of marijuana. *Journal of Clinical Pharmacology*, 42: 90S–96S.

Bruun, K., Pan, L. & Rexed, I. (1975). *The Gentlemen's Club: International Control of Drugs and Alcohol*. Chicago: University of Chicago Press.

Bryhni, A. (ed.) (2007). *Rusmidler i Norge – Alcohol and Drugs in Norway.* Oslo: SIRUS. http://www.sirus.no/files/pub/400/Rusmiddel%202007%20eng_web.pdf

Budney, A.J. & Hughes, J.R. (2006). The cannabis withdrawal syndrome. *Current Opinion in Psychiatry*, 19: 233–8.

Budney, A.J., Hughes, J.R., Moore, B.A. & Novy, P.L. (2001). Marijuana abstinence effects in marijuana smokers maintained in their home environment. *Archives of General Psychiatry*, 58: 917–24.

Budney, A.J., Hughes, J.R., Moore, B.A. & Vandrey, R. (2004). Review of the validity and significance of cannabis withdrawal syndrome. *American Journal of Psychiatry*, 161: 1967–77.

Budney, A.J., Vandrey, R.G., Hughes, J.R., Moore, B.A. & Bahrenburg, B. (2007). Oral delta-9-tetrahydrocannabinol suppresses cannabis withdrawal symptoms. *Drug and Alcohol Dependence*, 86: 22–9.

Bull, M. (2003). *Just Treatment: A Review of International Programs for the Diversion of Drug Related Offenders from the Criminal Justice System.* Department of the Premier and Cabinet Queensland: Queensland University of Technology.

Bull, M. (2005). A comparative review of best practice guidelines for the diversion of drug-related offenders. *International Journal of Drug Policy*, 16: 223–34.

Cabral, G.A. & Pettit, D.A.D. (1998). Drugs and immunity: Cannabinoids and their role in decreased resistance to infectious disease. *Journal of Neuroimmunology*, 83: 116–23.

Cadoni, C., Pisanu, A., Solinas, M., Acquas, E. & Di Chiara, G. (2001). Behavioural sensitization after repeated exposure to [Delta] 9-tetrahydrocannabinol and cross-sensitization with morphine. *Psychopharmacology*, 158: 259–66.

Cameron, L. & Williams, J. (2001) Cannabis, alcohol and cigarettes: Substitutes or complements? *Economic Record* 77: 19–34.

Cardoso, F.H. (2009) The war on drugs has failed. Now we need a more humane strategy. *Observer* (London), 6 September. http://www.guardian.co.uk/commentisfree/2009/sep/06/cardoso-war-on-drugs

Caspi, A., Moffitt, T.E., Cannon, M., McClay, J., Murray, R., Harrington, H., *et al.* (2005). Moderation of the effect of adolescent-onset cannabis use on adult psychosis by a functional polymorphism in the catechol-O-methyltransferase gene: Longitudinal evidence of a gene X environment interaction. *Biological Psychiatry*, 57: 1117–27.

Castle, D.J. & Murray, R.M. (eds.) (2004). *Marijuana and Madness: Psychiatry and Neurobiology.* Cambridge, UK: Cambridge University Press.

Castle, T. (2008). Cannabis classification to be tightened. In: *Reuters UK online, Wednesday May 7, 7:11BST.* http://uk.reuters.com/article/wtMostRead/idUKL0692965620080507?pageNumber=3&virtualBrandChannel=0&sp=true.

Caulkins, J. *et al.* (2005). *The Price of Illicit Drugs 1981–2003.* Santa Monica CA: RAND Corp.

Caulkins, J.P. (1999). Can supply factors suppress marijuana use by youth? *Drug Policy Analysis Bulletin* (Federation of American Scientists), 7: 3–5.

Caulkins, J.P. (2001). Comment on 'Should the DEA's STRIDE data be used for economic analysis of markets for illegal drugs?' *Journal of the American Statistical Association*, 96 (456): 1263–4.

Caulkins, J.P. & Pacula, R. (2006). Marijuana markets: Inferences from reports by the household population. *Journal of Drug Issues*, 36(1): 173–200.

Chambliss, W. (1975). *Criminal Law in Action.* Santa Barbara, CA: Hamilton Pub. Co.

Chang, L. & Chronicle, E.P. (2007). Functional imaging studies in cannabis users. *Neuroscientist*, 13: 422–32.

Charles, M., Bewley-Taylor, D. & Neidpath, A. (2005). *Drug Policy in India: Compounding Harm?* Beckley Park, Oxford, UK: Beckley Foundation, Briefing Paper 10. http://www.ahrn.net/library_upload/uploadfile/file2501.pdf

Chatwin, C. (2003). Drug policy developments within the European Union: The destabilizing effects of Dutch and Swedish drug policies. *British Journal of Criminology*, 43: 567–82.

Chatwin, C. (2007). Multi-level governance: The way forward for European illicit drug policy? *International Journal of Drug Policy*, 18: 494–502.

Chen, K. & Kandel, D.B. (1995). The natural history of drug use from adolescence to the mid-thirties in a general population sample. *American Journal of Public Health*, 85: 41–7.

Chesher, G. & Hall, W.D. (1999). Effects of cannabis on the cardiovascular and gastrointestinal systems. In: Kalant, H., Corrigall, W., Hall, W.D. & Smart, R. (eds.), *The Health Effects of Cannabis*. Toronto: Centre for Addiction and Mental Health, pp. 435–58.

Christie, P. & Ali, R. (2000). Offences under the Cannabis Expiation Notice Scheme in South Australia. *Drug and Alcohol Review*, 19(3): 251–6.

Clements, K.W. (2004). Three facts about marijuana prices. *Australian Journal of Agricultural & Resource Economics*, 48(2): 271–300.

Clements K.W. & Zhao X. (2005). *Economic Aspects of Marijuana*. Perth: University of Western Australia http://msc.uwa.edu.au/?f=148832

Coffey, C., Carlin, J. B., Degenhardt, L., Lynskey, M., Sanci, L. & Patton, G.C. (2002). Cannabis dependence in young adults: An Australian population study. *Addiction*, 97(2): 187–94.

Coffey, C., Carlin, J.B., Lynskey, M.T., Li, N. & Patton, G.C. (2003). Adolescent precursors of cannabis dependence: Findings from the Victorian Adolescent Health Cohort Study. *British Journal of Psychiatry*, 182: 330–6.

Cohen, S. (1976). The 94-day cannabis study. *Annals of the New York Academy of Sciences*, 282: 211–110.

Cohen, P. (1997). Crack in the Netherlands: Effective Social Policy is Effective Drug Policy. In: Reinarman, C. & Levine, H.G. (eds.), *Crack in America: Demon Drugs and Social Justice*. Berkeley: University of California Press, pp. 214–24.

Collin, C. (2006). *Substance Abuse Issues and Public Policy in Canada (1987–2005)*. Ottawa: Library of Parliament.

Collins, D. & Lapsley, H. (2007). *The Costs of Tobacco, Alcohol and Illicit Drug Use to Australian Society in 2004/05*. (National Drug Strategy Monograph 64). Canberra: Commonwealth Department of Health and Ageing. Available at: http://www.nationaldrugstrategy.gov.au/.

Collison, M. (1994). Drug crime, drug problems, and criminal justice: Sentencing trends and enforcement targets. *Howard Journal*, 33: 25–40.

Conforti, B. (1993). *International Law and the Role of Domestic Legal Systems*. Leiden: Martinus Nijhoff.

Copeland, J., Swift, W., Roffman, R. & Stephens, R. (2001). A randomized controlled trial of brief cognitive-behavioral interventions for cannabis use disorder. *Journal of Substance Abuse Treatment*, 21: 55–64.

Cornelius, M.D., Goldschmidt, L., Day, N.L. & Larkby, C. (2002). Alcohol, tobacco and marijuana use among pregnant teenagers: 6-year follow-up of offspring growth effects. *Neurotoxicology and Teratology*, 24: 703–10.

Costa, A.M. (2008). *Making drug control 'fit for purpose': Building on the UNGASS decade* Statement of the Executive Director of the United Nations Office on Drugs and Crime. http://www.unodc.org/documents/commissions/CND-Session51/CND-UNGASS-CRPs/ECN72008CRP17E.pdf

Council of Europe (1989). *Anti-Doping Convention*. Strasbourg: Council of Europe. http://conventions.coe.int/Treaty/Commun/QueVoulezVous.asp?NT=135&CM=8&CL=ENG

Council of Europe, Parliamentary Assembly (2007a). For a European convention promoting public health policy in the fight against drugs. Resolution 1576 (2007). Strasbourg: Council of Europe. http://assembly.coe.int/Main.asp?link=/Documents/AdoptedText/ta07/ERES1576.htm

Council of Europe, Parliamentary Assembly (2007b). For a European drug convention on promoting public health policy in drug control, Doc. 11344, 10 July 2007. Report, Social, Health and Family Affairs Committee. (http://assembly.coe.int/Main.asp?link=/Documents/WorkingDocs/Doc07/EDOC11344.htm)

D'Souza, D.C. (2007). Cannabinoids and psychosis. *International Review of Neurobiology*, 78: 289–326.

D'Souza, D.C., Abi-Saab, W.M., Madonick, S., Forselius-Bielen, K., Doersch, A., Braley, G., *et al.* (2005). Delta-9-tetrahydrocannabinol effects in schizophrenia: Implications for cognition, psychosis, and addiction. *Biological Psychiatry*, 57: 594–608.

D'Souza, D.C., Cho, H.S., Perry, E. & Krystal, J.H. (2004). Cannabinoid 'model' psychosis, dopamine-cannabinoid interactions and implications for schizophrenia. In: Castle, D.J. & Murray, R.M. (eds.), *Marijuana and Madness*. Cambridge, UK: Cambridge University Press, pp. 142–65.

Day, N.L., Wagener, D. & Taylor, P. (1985). Measurement of substance use during pregnancy: Methodologic issues. In: Pinkert, T. (ed.), *Current Research on the Consequences of Maternal Drug Abuse*. Rockville, MD: U. S. Department of Health and Human Services, pp. 36–47.

Day, N.L., Richardson, G.A., Goldschmidt, L., Robles, N., Taylor, P.M., Stoffer, D.S., *et al.* (1994). Effect of prenatal marijuana exposure on the cognitive development of offspring at age three. *Neurotoxicology and Teratology*, 16: 169–75.

de Kort, M. & Cramer, T. (1999). Pragmatism versus ideology: Dutch drug policy continued. *Journal of Drug Issues*, 29: 473–93.

de Matons, J.G. (2004). *Facilitation of Transport and Trade in Sub-Saharan Africa: A Review of International Legal Instruments*. Washington: World Bank, Sub-Saharan African Transport Policy Program, SSATP Working Paper No. 73. http://www4.worldbank.org/afr/ssatp/Resources/HTML/legal_review/Main%20Texts/SSATPWP73.pdf

de Preux, E., Dubois-Arber, F. & Zobel, F. (2004). Current trends in illegal drug use and drug related health problems in Switzerland. *Swiss Medical Weekly*, 134: 313–21.

de Zwart, W. & van Laar, M. (2001). Cannabis regimes. *British Journal of Psychiatry*, 178: 574–5.

Degenhardt, L. & Hall, W.D. (2001). The association between psychosis and problematical drug use among Australian adults: Findings from the National Survey of Mental Health and Well-being. *Psychological Medicine*, 31: 659–68.

Degenhardt, L. & Hall, W.D. (2006). Is cannabis a contributory cause of psychosis? *Canadian Journal of Psychiatry*, 51: 556–65.

Degenhardt, L., Hall, W.D. & Lynskey, M. (2000). Cohort trends in the age of initiation of drug use in Australia. *Australian and New Zealand Journal of Public Health*, 24: 421–6.

Degenhardt, L., Hall, W.D. & Lynskey, M.T. (2003). Testing hypotheses about the relationship between cannabis use and psychosis. *Drug and Alcohol Dependence*, 71: 37–48.

Degenhardt, L., Chiu, W.T., Sampson, N., Kessler, R.C., Anthony, J.C., *et al.* (2008). Toward a global view of alcohol, tobacco, cannabis, and cocaine use: Findings from the WHO World Mental Health Surveys. *PLOS Medicine* 5(7): e141 http://medicine. plosjournals.org/perlserv/?request=get-document&doi=10.1371/journal.pmed.0050141

Denis, C., Lavie, E., Fatseas, M. & Auriacombe, M. (2006). Psychotherapeutic interventions for cannabis abuse and/or dependence in outpatient settings. *Cochrane Database of Systematic Reviews*, 3: CD005336.

DiFranco, M., Sheppard, H., Hunter, D., Tosteson , T. & Ascher, M. (1996). The lack of association of marijuana and other recreational drugs with progression to AIDS in the San Francisco Men's Health Study. *Annals of Epidemiology*, 6: 283–9.

Donnelly, N. & Hall, W. (1994). *Patterns of Cannabis Use in Australia. National Drug Strategy.* [27]. Canberra: Australian Government Printing Service.

Donnelly, N., Hall, W. & Christie, P. (1999). *The Effects of the CEN Scheme on Levels and Patterns of Cannabis Use In South Australia: Evidence from National Drug Strategy Household Surveys 1985–1995.* Canberra: Commomwealth Department of Health and Family Services.

Donnelly, N., Hall, W. & Christie, P. (2000). The effects of the Cannabis Expiation Notice scheme on levels and patterns of cannabis use in South Australia: Evidence from National Drug Strategy Household Surveys 1985–95. *Drug and Alcohol Review*, 19(3): 265–9.

Donnelly, N., Oldenburg, B., Quine, S., Macaskill, P., Flaherty, B., Spooner, C. & Lyle, D. (1992). Changes reported in drug prevalence among New South Wales secondary school students 1983–1989. *Australian Journal of Public Health*, 16(1): 50–7.

Donovan, J.E. & Jessor, R. (1983). Problem drinking and the dimension of involvement with drugs: A Guttman scalogram analysis of adolescent drug use. *American Journal of Public Health*, 73: 543–52.

Donovan, J.E. & Jessor, R. (1985). Structure of problem behavior in adolescence and young adulthood. *Journal of Consulting and Clinical Psychology*, 53: 890–904.

Dorn, N. (2004). UK policing of drug traffickers and users: Policy implementation in the context of national law, European traditions, international drug conventions, and security after 2001. *Journal of Drug Issues*, 34: 533–50.

Draper, G. & Serafino, S. (2006). *2004 National Drug Strategy Household Survey Western Australia results.* Perth: Epidemiology Branch, Department of Health WA Drug and Alcohol Office.

Drug and Alcohol Office (2007a). *Statutory Review of Cannabis Control Act 2003. Report to the Minister for Health: Executive Summary.* Perth, Western Australia: Drug and Alcohol Office.

Drug and Alcohol Office. (2007b). *Statutory Review of Cannabis Control Act 2003. Report to the Minister for Health: Technical Report.* Perth, Western Australia: Drug and Alcohol Office.

Drug War Chronicle (2006). Brazilian President signs new drug law – No jail for users. *Drug War Chronicle,* Issue 451, Sept. 1. http://stopthedrugwar.org/chronicle/451/lula_signs_new_brazil_drug_law_no_jail_for_users

Drug War Chronicle (2008). Brazil Appeals Court Rules Drug Possession Not a Crime. *Drug War Chronicle,* Issue 538, May 30. http://stopthedrugwar.org/chronicle/538/brazil_appeals_court_drug_possession_no_crime

Drummer, O.H., Gerostamoulos, J., Batziris, H., Chu, M., Caplehorn, J., Robertson, M.D., *et al.* (2004). The involvement of drugs in drivers of motor vehicles killed in Australian road traffic crashes. *Accident Analysis and Prevention,* 36: 239–48.

Duncan, D. & Nicholson, T. (1997). Dutch drug policy: A model for America? *Journal of Health and Social Policy,* 8: 1–15.

Duncan, S.C., Duncan, T.E., Biglan, A. & Ary, D. (1998). Contributions of the social context to the development of adolescent substance use: A multivariate latent growth modeling approach. *Drug and Alcohol Dependence,* 50: 57–71.

Dutch National Alcohol and Drug Information System (2006). Treatment demand of cannabis users 2004). *LADIS News Flash,* pp. 1–2. Houten, Netherlands: Stichting IVZ. http://www.sivz.nl/content/_files/LADIS_News_Flash_cannabis.pdf?PHPSESSID=45d9 d62d34f12464355f35e3f68455dd

Edwards, G. (2005). *Matters of Substance—Drugs: Is Legalization the Right Answer – or the Wrong Question?* London, etc.: Penguin Books.

Eidgennossische Kommission für Drogenfragen (2008). *Cannabis 2008: Lagenbeurteilung und Empfehlungen der Eidgenossischen Kommission fur Drogenfragen.* Berne: Eidgennossische Kommission für Drogenfragen.

Ellickson, P., Bui, K., Bell, R. & McGuigan, K.A. (1998). Does early drug use increase the risk of dropping out of high school? *Journal of Drug Issues,* 28: 357–80.

Ellison, E. (2004). Policing cannabis: Can pragmatism replace policy? *Probation Journal,* 51: 415–20.

ElSohly, M.A. (2002). Chemical constituents of cannabis. In: Grotenhermen, F. & Russo, E. (eds.), *Cannabis and Cannabinoids: Pharmacology, Toxicology and Therapeutic Potential.* London: Haworth.

ElSohly, M.A. (2008). *Quarterly Report: December 16, 2007 thru March 15, 2008.* (Potency Monitoring Project Report 100). University, MS: National Center for Natural Products Research, University of Mississippi.

ElSohly, M.A., Ross, S.A., Mehmedic, Z., Arafat, R., Yi, B. & Banahan, B.F. (2000). Potency trends of delta(9)-THC and other cannabinoids in confiscated marijuana from 1980–1997. *Journal of Forensic Sciences,* 45: 24–30.

EMCDDA (2003). *Annual Report 2003: The State of the Drugs Problem in the European Union and Norway.* Luxembourg: Office for Official Publications of the European Communities. Available at: http://candidates2003.emcdda.europa.eu/en/home-en.html.

EMCDDA (2004a). *An Overview of Cannabis Potency in Europe.* Insights, No. 6. Lisbon: EMCDDA. http://www.emcdda.europa.eu/html.cfm/index33984EN.html

EMCDDA (2004b). 'Cannabis problems in context – understanding the increase in European treatment demands'. Chapter from: *Annual report on the state of the drugs problem in the European Union and Norway.* Lisbon: EMCDDA.

EMCDDA (2005). *Thematic Papers: Illicit Drug Use in the EU: Legislative Approaches.* Lisbon: European Monitoring Centre for Drugs and Drug Addiction. eldd.emcdda. europa.eu/attachements.cfm/att_10080_EN_EMCDDATP_01.pdf

EMCDDA (2006). *Annual Report 2006: The State of the Drugs Problem in Europe.* Lisbon: European Monitoring Centre for Drugs and Drug Addiction.

EMCDDA (2007a). *Annual Report 2007: The State Of The Drugs Problem in Europe* Lisbon: EMCDDA.

EMCDDA (2007b). *European Legal Database on Drugs – Topic Overviews*– Possession of cannabis for personal use. Lisbon: European Monitoring Centre for Drugs and Drug Addiction. http://eldd.emcdda.europa.eu/html.cfm/index5769EN.html

EMCDDA (2007c). *Statistical Bulletin 2007.* Lisbon: European Monitoring Centre for Drugs and Drug Addiction. http://www.emcdda.europa.eu/html.cfm/ index34943EN.html

EMCDDA (2007d). *Annual Report 2007: The State Of The Drugs Problem in Europe.* Lisbon: EMCDDA.

ENCOD (2009a). Cannabis Social Clubs. Antwerp: European Coalition for Just and Effective Drug Polliies (ENCOD). http://www.encod.org/info/-CANNABIS-SOCIAL-CLUBS-.html

ENCOD (2009b). Pannagh, Spain. Antwerp: European Coalition for Just and Effective Drug PolIcies (ENCOD). http://www.encod.org/info/PANNAGH-SPAIN.html

English, D., Hulse, G., Milne, E., Holman, C. & Bower, C. (1997). Maternal cannabis use and birth weight: A meta-analysis. *Addiction*, 92: 1553–60.

Erickson, P. (1976). Deterrence and deviance: The example of cannabis prohibition. *The Journal of Criminal Law and Criminology*, 67(2): 222–32.

Erickson, P. (1980). *Cannabis Criminals: The Social Effects of Punishment on Drug Users.* Toronto: Addiction Research Foundation.

Erickson, P. & Murray, G. (1986). Cannabis criminals revisited. *British Journal of Addiction*, 81: 81–5.

Erickson, P. & Oscapella, E. (1999). Cannabis in Canada – A puzzling policy. *International Journal of Drug Policy*, 10: 313–18.

Ericson, R. & Baranek, P. (1982). *The Ordering Of Justice: A Study of Accused Persons as Dependants in the Criminal Process.* Toronto: University of Toronto Press.

European Legal Database on Drugs (2004a). *Country Profile–Austria.* http://eldd.emcdda. europa.eu/html.cfm/index5174EN.html

European Legal Database on Drugs (2004b). *Country Profile–France.* http://eldd.emcdda. europa.eu/index.cfm?fuseaction=public.content&sLanguageISO=EN&nNodeID=5174

Eyler, F.D. & Behnke, M. (1999). Early development of infants exposed to drugs prenatally. *Clinics in Perinatology*, 26: 107–50.

Fankhauser, W. (2008). Cannabis as medicine in Europe in the 19th Century. In: Rödner Sznitman, S., Olsson, B. & Room, R. (eds.) *A Cannabis Reader: Global Issues and Local Experiences.* vol. 1, pp. 5–14. Lisbon, European Monitoring Center on Drugs and Drug Abuse. http://www.emcdda.europa.eu/publications/monographs/ cannabis

Farrelly, M.C., Bray, J.W., Zarkin, G.A. & Wendling, B.W. (2001). The joint demand for cigarettes and marijuana: Evidence from the National Household Surveys on Drug Abuse. *Journal of Health Economics*, 20: 51–68.

Fergusson, D.M., Lynskey, M.T. & Horwood, L.J. (1996). The short-term consequences of early onset cannabis use. *Journal of Abnormal Child Psychology*, 24: 499–512.

Fergusson, D.M. & Horwood, L.J. (1997). Early onset cannabis use and psychosocial adjustment in young adults. *Addiction*, 92: 279–96.

Fergusson, D.M. & Horwood, L.J. (2000). Does cannabis use encourage other forms of illicit drug use? *Addiction*, 95: 505–20.

Fergusson, D.M. & Horwood, L.J. (2001). Cannabis use and traffic accidents in a birth cohort of young adults. *Accident Analysis and Prevention*, 33: 703–11.

Fergusson, D.M., Horwood, L.J. & Northstone, K. (2002a). Maternal use of cannabis and pregnancy outcome. *British Journal of Obstetrics and Gynaecology*, 109: 21–7.

Fergusson, D.M., Horword, L.J. & Swain-Campbell, N. (2002b). Cannabis use and psychosocial adjustment in adolescence and young adulthood. *Addiction*, 97: 1123–35.

Fergusson, D.M., Horwood, L.J. & Swain-Campbell, N.R. (2003). Cannabis dependence and psychotic symptoms in young people. *Psychological Medicine*, 33: 15–21.

Fetherston, J. & Lenton, S. (2007). *A Pre-Post Comparison of the Impacts of the Western Australian Cannabis Infringement Notice Scheme on Public Attitudes, Knowledge and Use*. Perth: National Drug Research Institute, Curtin University of Technology.

Fischer, B., Room, R. & Ala-Leppilampi, K. (2001). Cannabis-use control in western countries – A brief review of history and present. In: European City Conference on Cannabis Policy (conference book), pp. 37–42. The Hague: ES&E.

Fischer, B., Ala-Leppilampi, K., Single, E. & Robins, A. (2003). Cannabis law reform in Canada: Is the 'saga of promise, hesitation and retreat' coming to an end? *Canadian Journal of Criminology and Criminal Justice*, 45(3): 265–97.

Fitzsimmons, G. & Cooper-Stanbury, M. (2000). *1998 National Drug Strategy Household Survey – State and Territory Results*. Canberra: Australian Institute of Health and Welfare.

Forrester, M.B. & Merz, R.D. (2007). Risk of selected birth defects with prenatal illicit drug use, Hawaii, 1986–2002. *Journal of Toxicology and Environmental Health Part A*, 70: 7–18.

Fosados, R., Evans, E. & Hser, Y. (2007). Ethnic difference in utilization of drug treatment services and outcomes among Proposition 36 offenders in California. *Journal of Substance Abuse Treatment*, 33: 391–9.

Fosdick, R.B. and Scott, A.L. (1933). *Toward Liquor Control*. New York: Harper & Brothers Publishers.

Fratello, D. (2006). *Proposition 36: Improving Lives, Delivering Results – A Review of the First Four Years of California's Substance Abuse and Crime Prevention Act of 2000*. San Francisco: Drug Policy Alliance.

Fried, P.A. & Smith, A.R. (2001). A literature review of the consequences of prenatal marihuana exposure: An emerging theme of a deficiency in aspects of executive function. *Neurotoxicology and Teratology*, 23: 1–11.

Fried, P.A. & Watkinson, B. (2000). Visuoperceptual functioning differs in 9- to 12-year olds prenatally exposed to cigarettes and marihuana. *Neurotoxicology and Teratology*, 22: 11–20.

Gable, R.S. (2004). Comparison of acute lethal toxicity of commonly abused psychoactive substances. *Addiction*, 99: 686–96.

Gamella, J.F. & Jiménez Rodrigo, M.L. (2004). A brief history of cannabis policies in Spain (1968–2003). *Journal of Drug Issues,* 623–59.

Gamella, J.F. & Jiménez Rodrigo, M.L. (2008). Multinational export–import ventures: Moroccan hashish into Europe through Spain. In: Rödner Sznitman, S., Olsson, B. & Room, R. (eds.). *A Cannabis Reader: Global Issues and Local Experiences*, vol. 1, pp. 261–89. Lisbon, European Monitoring Center on Drugs and Drug Abuse. http://www.emcdda.europa.eu/publications/monographs/cannabis

Gardner, E. (1999). Cannabinoid interaction with brain reward systems. In: Nahas, G.G., Sutin, K., Harvey, D. & Agurell, S. (eds.), *Marihuana and Medicine*. Totowa, NJ: Humana Press, pp. 187–205.

Geiser, U. (2007). Pot smokers hope for support in parliament. Bern: Swissinfo. http://www.swissinfo.org/eng/politics/internal_affairs/Pot_smokers_hope_for_support_in_parliament.html?siteSect=1511&sid=8469963&cKey=1197372388000&ty=st

Gelders, D. & Vander Laenen, F. (2007). Mr. Police Officer I thought cannabis was legal; introducing new policy regarding cannabis in Belgium: A story of good intentions and Babel. *Drugs: Education, Prevention & Policy*, 14: 103–16.

Gerberich, S.G., Sidney, S., Braun, B.L., Tekawa, I.S., Tolan, K.K. & Quesenberry, C.P. (2003). Marijuana use and injury events resulting in hospitalization. *Annals of Epidemiology*, 13: 230–7.

Gettman, J. (2007). Lost taxes and other costs of marijuana laws. Report for the *Bulletin of Cannabis Reform* http://www.drugscience.org/Archive/bcr4/bcr4_index.html

Gibson, G., Baghurst, P. & Colley, D. (1983). Maternal alcohol, tobacco and cannabis consumption and the outcome of pregnancy. *Australian and New Zealand Journal of Obstetrics and Gynaecology*, 23: 15–19.

Giffen, J., Endicott, S. & Lambert, S. (1991). *Panic and Indifference – The Politics of Canada's Drug Laws*. Ottawa: Canadian Centre on Substance Abuse.

Goldkamp, J., White, M. & Robinson, J. (2001). Do drug courts work? Getting inside the drug court black box. *Journal of Drug Issues*, 31: 27–72.

Goldschmidt, L., Day, N.L. & Richardson, G.A. (2000). Effects of prenatal marijuana exposure on child behavior problems at age 10. *Neurotoxicology and Teratology*, 22: 325–36.

Golub, A. & Johnson, B. (2001). Variation in youthful risks of progression from alcohol and tobacco to marijuana and to hard drugs across generations. *American Journal of Public Health*, 91(2): 225–32.

Golub, A., Johnson, B.D. & Dunlap, E. (2007). The race/ethnicity disparity in misdemeanor marijuana arrests in New York City. *Criminology & Public Policy*, 6(1): 301–35.

Gottfredson, D. (1987). Prediction and classification in criminal justice decision making. *Crime & Justice*, 9: 1–20.

Gottschalk, L., Aronow, W. & Prakash, R. (1977). Effect of marijuana and placebo-marijuana smoking on psychological state and on psychophysiological and cardiovascular functioning in angina patients. *Biological Psychiatry*, 12: 255–66.

Gouyis Roman, C., Ahn-Redding, H. & Simon, R.J. (2005). *Illicit Drug Policies, Trafficking, and Use the World Over*. Lanham, MD & Plymouth, UK: Lexington Books.

Greenfield, T.K., Kerr, W.C., Bond, J., Ye, Y. & Stockwell, T. (forthcoming). Improving graduated frequencies alcohol measures for monitoring consumption patterns: Results from US and Australian national surveys and a diary validity study. *Contemporary Drug Problems*.

Greenfield, T.K. & Rogers, J.D. (1999). Who drinks most of the alcohol in the U.S.? The policy implications. *Journal of Studies on Alcohol*, 60(1): 78–89.

Grossman, M. (2005). Individual behaviors and substance use: The role of price, in: Lindgren, B. & Grossman, M. (eds.) *Substance Use: Individual Behaviors, Social Interactions, Markets and Politics*, Advances in Health Economics and Health Services Research Vol. 16, Amsterdam: Elsevier. http://ideas.repec.org/p/nbr/nberwo/10948.html

Grotenhermen, F. (2007). The toxicology of cannabis and cannabis prohibition. *Chemistry & Biodiversity*, 4: 1744–69.

Grotenhermen, F., Leson, G., Berghaus, G., Drummer, O.H., Kruger, H.P., Longo, M., *et al.* (2007). Developing limits for driving under cannabis. *Addiction*, 102: 1910–17.

Grufferman, S., Schwartz, A.G., Ruymann, F.B. & Maurer, H.M. (1993). Parents' use of cocaine and marijuana and increased risk of rhabdomyosarcoma in their children. *Cancer Causes and Control*, 4: 217–24.

Gurney, J., Smith, M.A. & Bunin, C. (2000a). CNS and miscellaneous intracranial and intraspinal neoplasms. In: Reis, L., Eisner, M., Kosary, C., Hankey, B., Miller, B., Clegg, L., *et al.* (eds.), *SEER Cancer Statistics Review, 1973–1997*. Bethesda, MD: National Cancer Institute, pp. 51–63.

Gurney, J., Young, J., Roffers, S., Smith, M.A. & Bunin, C. (2000b). Soft tissue sarcomas. In: Reis, L., Eisner, M., Kosary, C., Hankey, B., Miller, B., Clegg, L., *et al.* (eds.), *SEER Cancer Statistics Review, 1973–1997*. Bethesda, MD: National Cancer Institute, pp. 11–123.

Haden, M. (2004). Regulation of illegal drugs: An exploration of public health tools. *International Journal of Drug Policy* 15: 225–30.

Hakkarainen, P., Kainulainen, H. & Perälä, J. (2008). Measuring the cannabis market in Finland: A consumption-based estimate. *Contemporary Drug Problems*, 35: 321–46.

Hales, J., Mayne, M., Swan, A., Alberti, S. & Ritter, A. (2004). *Evaluation of Queensland Illicit Drug Diversion Initiative (QIDDI) Police Diversion Program: Final Report* Brisbane: Queensland Health.

Hall, W.D. (1995). The public health significance of cannabis use in Australia. *Australian Journal of Public Health*, 19: 235–42.

Hall, W.D. (1999). Assessing the health and psychological effects of cannabis use. In: Kalant, H., Corrigall, W., Hall, W.D. & Smart, R. (eds.), *The Health Effects of Cannabis*. Toronto: Centre for Addiction and Mental Health, pp. 1–17.

Hall, W.D. (2008). The contribution of research to the development of a national cannabis policy in Australia. *Addiction*, 103: 712–20.

Hall, W. & Degenhardt, L. (2003). Medical marijuana initiatives: Are they justified? How successful are they likely to be? *CNS Drugs*, 17: 689–97.

Hall, W.D., Degenhardt, L. & Lynskey, M.T. (2001). *The Health and Psychological Effects of Cannabis Use*. (National Drug Strategy Monograph 44). Canberra: Commonwealth Department of Health and Aged Care. Available at: http://www.health.gov.au.

Hall, W.D., Degenhardt, L. & Sindicich, N. (2008b in press). Illicit drug use and the burden of disease. In: Heggenhougen, K. & Quah, S. (eds.), *International Encyclopedia of Public Health*. Amsterdam: Elsevier.

Hall, W.D., Doran, C., Degenhardt, L. & Shepard, D. (2006). Illicit opioid dependence. In: Jamison, D., Evans, D. & Alleyne, G. (eds.), *Disease Control Priorities for Developing Countries*. New York: Oxford University Press, pp. 907–31.

Hall, W.D. & Lynskey, M.T. (2005). Is cannabis a gateway drug? Testing hypotheses about the relationship between cannabis use and the use of other illicit drugs. *Drug and Alcohol Review*, 24: 39–48.

Hall, W.D., Room, R. & Bondy, S. (1999). Comparing the health and psychological risks of alcohol, cannabis, nicotine and opiate use. In: Kalant, H., Corrigal, W., Hall, W.D. & Smart, R. (eds.), *The Health Effects of Cannabis*. Toronto: Centre for Addiction and Mental Health, pp. 475–506.

Hall, W.D. & MacPhee, D. (2002). Cannabis use and cancer. *Addiction*, 97: 243–7.

Hall, W.D. and Pacula, R.L. (2003). *Cannabis Use and Dependence: Public Health and Public Policy*. Cambridge, etc.: Cambridge University Press.

Hall, W.D. & Solowij, N. (1998). The adverse effects of cannabis use. *Lancet*, 352: 1611–16.

Hall, W.D. & Swift, W. (2000). The THC content of cannabis in Australia: Evidence and implications. *Australian and New Zealand Journal of Public Health*, 24: 503–08.

Han, C., McGue, M.K. & Iacono, W.G. (1999). Lifetime tobacco, alcohol and other substance use in adolescent Minnesota twins: Univariate and multivariate behavioral genetic analyses. *Addiction*, 94: 981–93.

Harris, A. (2005). *Consumer Trends No. 36: Quarter 1, 2005*. London: Office of National Statistics. http://www.statistics.gov.uk/downloads/theme_economy/CT2005Q1.pdf

Hart, C.L. (2005). Increasing treatment options for cannabis dependence: A review of potential pharmacotherapies. *Drug and Alcohol Dependence*, 80: 147–59.

Hashibe, M., Straif, K., Tashkin, D.P., Morgenstern, H., Greenland, S. & Zhang, Z.F. (2005). Epidemiologic review of marijuana use and cancer risk. *Alcohol*, 35: 265–75.

Hatch, E. & Bracken, M. (1986). Effect of marijuana use in pregnancy on fetal growth. *American Journal of Epidemiology*, 124: 986–93.

Hawkins, J.D., Catalano, R.F. & Miller, J.Y. (1992). Risk and protective factors for alcohol and other drug problems in adolescence and early adulthood: Implications for substance abuse prevention. *Psychological Bulletin*, 112: 64–105.

Heale, P., Hawks, D. & Lenton, S. (2000). Public awareness, knowledge and attitudes regarding the CEN System in South Australia. *Drug and Alcohol Review*, 19(3): 271–80.

Health Canada (2005). *Medical Use of Marihuana – FAQs*. Ottawa: Health Canada. http://www.hc-sc.gc.ca/dhp-mps/marihuana/about-apropos/faq-eng.php

Heath, A.C. (1995). Genetic influences on alcoholism risk: A review of adoption and twin studies. *Alcohol Health and Research World*, 19: 166–71.

Helfer, L.R. (2005). Exiting treaties. *Virginia Law Review*, 91: 1579–648. http://ssrn.com/abstract=683481

Helfer, L.R. (2006). Not fully committed? Reservations, risk and treaty design. *Yale Journal of International Law*, 31: 367–82. http://www.yale.edu/yjil/PDFs/vol_31/Helfer.pdf

Hendrick, D., Martin, M. & Greenberg, P. (2003). *Conditional Sentencing in Canada: A Statisical Profile 1997–2001*. Report 85-560-XIE.

Henquet, C., Krabbendam, L., de Graaf, R., ten Have, M. & van Os, J. (2006). Cannabis use and expression of mania in the general population. *Journal of Affective Disorders*, 95: 103–10.

Henquet, C., Krabbendam, L., Spauwen, J., Kaplan, C., Lieb, R., Wittchen, H.U., *et al.* (2004). Prospective cohort study of cannabis use, predisposition for psychosis, and psychotic symptoms in young people. *BMJ*, 330: 11.

Heustis, M.A. (2005). Pharmacokinetics and metabolism of the plant cannabinoids, delta9-tetrahydrocannabinol, cannabidiol and cannabinol. *Handbook of Experimental Pharmacology*, 168: 657–90.

Heustis, M.A., Gorelick, D.A., Heishman, S.J., Preston, K.L., Nelson, R.A., Moochan, E.T., *et al.* (2001). Blockade of effects of smoked marijuana by the CB1-selective cannabinoid receptor antagonist SR141716. *Archives of General Psychiatry*, 58: 322–8.

Hibell, B., Andersson, B., Bjarnason, T., Ahlström, S., Balakireva, O., Kokkevi, A. & Morgan, M. (2004). *The ESPAD Report 2003: Alcohol and Other Drug Use Among Students in 35 European Countries*. Stockholm: Swedish Council for Information on Alcohol and Other Drugs.

Hickman, M., Vickerman, P., Macleod, J., Kirkbride, J. & Jones, P.B. (2007). Cannabis and schizophrenia: Model projections of the impact of the rise in cannabis use on historical and future trends in schizophrenia in England and Wales. *Addiction*, 102: 597–606.

Hillman, S.D., Silburn, S.R., Green, A. & Zubrick, S.R. (2000). *Youth Suicide in Western Australia Involving Cannabis and Other Drugs*. Perth: Western Australian Drug Abuse Strategy Office.

Hilts, P.H. (1994). Is nicotine addictive? It depends on whose criteria you use: Experts say the definition of addiction is evolving. *New York Times* 2 August: p. C3.

Hingson, R., Alpert, J., Day, N., Dooling, E., Kayne, H., Morelock, S., *et al.* (1982a). Effects of maternal drinking and marijuana use on fetal growth and development. *Pediatrics*, 70: 539–46.

Hingson, R., Heeren, T., Mangione, T., Morelock, S. & Mucatel, M. (1982b). Teenage driving after using marijuana or drinking and traffic accident involvement. *Journal of Safety Research*, 13: 33–7.

Holder, H.D. & Cherpitel, C.J. (1996). The end of U.S. prohibition: A case study of Mississippi. *Contemporary Drug Problems* 23(2): 301–30.

Hollister, L.E. (1986). Health aspects of cannabis. *Pharmacological Reviews*, 38: 1–20.

House of Commons of Canada (2004). *Bill C-17*. Ottawa: Minister of Justice. http://www2.parl.gc.ca/HousePublications/Publication.aspx?Docid=2333887&file=4 [accessed June 23, 2008]

Hughes, C.E. & Stevens, A. (2007). *The Effects of Decriminalization of Drug Use in Portugal, Briefing Paper14*. London: The Beckley Foundation Drug Policy Program.

Huizink, A.C. & Mulder, E.J. (2006). Maternal smoking, drinking or cannabis use during pregnancy and neurobehavioral and cognitive functioning in human offspring. *Neuroscience and Biobehavioral Reviews*, 30: 24–41.

Hutchings, D. & Fried, P.A. (1999). Cannabis during pregnancy: Neurobehavioural effects in animals and humans. In: Kalant, H., Corrigall, W., Hall, W.D. & Smart, R. (eds.), *The Health Effects of Cannabis*. Toronto: Centre for Addiction and Mental Health, pp. 435–58.

IDPC (2007). *The 2007 Commission on Narcotic Drugs.* IDPC Briefing Paper No. 5. Witley, Surrey, UK: International Drug Policy Consortium. http://www. internationaldrugpolicy.net/reports/IDPC_Report_5.pdf

INCB (2007). *Report of the International Narcotics Control Board for 2006.* New York: United Nations. http://www.incb.org/pdf/e/ar/2006/annual-report-2006-en.pdf

INCB (2008). *Report of the International Narcotics Control Board for 2007.* New York: United Nations. http://www.incb.org/incb/annual-report-2007.html

Iulianelli, L.A., Guanabara, L.P., Fraga, P.C.P. & T. Blickman (2004). *A Pointles War: Drugs and Violence in Brazil,* Amsterdam: TransNational Institute.

Iversen, L. (2007). *The Science of Marijuana.* Oxford: Oxford University Press.

Jenkins, S. (2009) The war on drugs is immoral idiocy. We need the courage of Argentina. *Guardian* (London), 3 September. http://www.guardian.co.uk/commentisfree/2009/sep/03/drugs-prohibition-latin-america

Johnson, B., Dunlap, E., Sifaneckl, S.J. & Ream, G.L. (2007). *Ethnicity, Marijuana Use Etiquette, and Marijuana-Related Police Contact in New York City.* Presented at the annual meeting of the American Sociological Association, New York City. http://www.allacademic.com/meta/p_mla_apa_research_citation/1/8/2/9/4/p182943_index.html

Johnston, L. D., O'Malley, P. M. & Bachman, J. G. (1981). *Marijuana decriminalisation: The impact on Youth1975-80. Monitoring the Future. Occasional Paper Series. Paper 13.* Ann Arbor: Institute for Social Research, Michigan University.

Johnston, L.D., O'Malley, P.M., Bachman, J.G. & Schulenberg, J.E. (2007). *Monitoring the Future National Survey Results on Drug Use, 1975–2006: Volume I, Secondary School Students* (NIH Publication No. 07-6205). Bethesda, MD: National Institute on Drug Abuse.

Jones, R.T. (2002). Cardiovascular system effects of marijuana. *Journal of Clinical Pharmacology*, 42: 58S–63S.

Jones, R.T., Benowitz, N. & Herning, R.I. (1976). The 30-day trip: Clinical studies of cannabis use, tolerance and dependence. In: Braude, M. & Szara, S. (eds.), *The Pharmacology of Marijuana.* New York: Academic Press, Vol. 2, pp. 627–42.

Joy, J., Watson, S. & Benson, J. (eds.) (1999). *Marijuana and Medicine -- Assessing the Science Base.* A report of the Institute of Medicine. Washington D.C: National Academy Press.

Justice Research and Statistics Association (2000). *Creating a New Criminal Justice System for the 21st Century: Findings and Results from State and Local Program Evaluations.* Washington DC: US Bureau of Justice Assistance.

Kalant, H. (2004). Adverse effects of cannabis on health: An update of the literature since 1996. *Progress in Neuro-Psychopharmacology and Biological Psychiatry*, 28: 849–63.

Kalant, H., Corrigal, W., Hall, W.D. & Smart, R. (eds.) (1999). *The Health Effects of Cannabis.* Toronto: Centre for Addiction and Mental Health.

Kandel, D.B. (1984). Marijuana users in young adulthood. *Archives of General Psychiatry*, 41: 200–09.

Kandel, D.B. (2002). *Stages and Pathways of Drug Involvement: Examining the Gateway Hypothesis.* New York: Cambridge University Press.

Kandel, D.B., Davies, M., Karus, D. & Yamaguchi, K. (1986). The consequences in young adulthood of adolescent drug involvement: An overview. *Archives of General Psychiatry*, 43: 746–54.

Kandel, D.B. & Davies, M. (1992). Progression to regular marijuana involvement: Phenomenology and risk factors for near-daily use. In: M. Glantz & R. Pickens (eds.), *Vulnerability to Drug Abuse* (pp. 211–53). Washington, DC: American Psychological Association.

Kapp, C. (2003). Swiss debate whether to legalise cannabis. *The Lancet*, 362: 970–71.

Kaslow, R.A., Blackwelder, W.C., Ostrow, D.G., Yerg, D., Palenicek, J., Coulson, A.H., *et al.* (1989). No evidence for a role of alcohol or other psychoactive drugs in accelerating immunodeficiency in HIV–1-positive individuals: A report from the Multicenter AIDS Cohort Study. *JAMA*, 261: 3424–9.

Kellough, G. & Wortley, S. (2002). Remand for plea: Bail decisions and plea bargaining as commensurate decisions. *British Journal of Criminology*, 42: 186–210.

Kelly, E., Darke, S. & Ross, J. (2004). A review of drug use and driving: Epidemiology, impairment, risk factors and risk perceptions. *Drug and Alcohol Review*, 23: 319–44.

Kessler, D. & Piehl, A. (1998). The role of discretion in the criminal justice system. *Journal of Law, Economics, and Organization*, 14: 256–76.

Kessler, R.C., McGonagle, K.A., Zhao, S., Nelson, C.B., Hughes, M., Eshleman, S., *et al.* (1994). Lifetime and 12-month prevalence of DSM-III-R psychiatric disorders in the United States. Results from the National Comorbidity Survey. *Archives of General Psychiatry*, 51: 8–19.

Khatapoush, S. & Hallfors, D. (2004). Sending the wrong message: did medical marijuana legalization in California change attitudes about use of marijuana? *Journal of Drug Issues*, 34: 751–70.

Kilmer, B. (2002). Do cannabis possession laws influence cannabis use? In: *Cannabis 2002 Report – Technical Report of the International Scientific Conference, Brussels, Belgium* (pp. 101–23). Brussels: Ministry of Public Health of Belgium.

Kilmer, B. & R. Pacula (2009). *Estimating the Size of Global Drug Market Revenues*. Report to the European Commission, Directorate-General for Justice, Freedom and Security (Jls/2007/C4/005

Kleber, H.D., Weiss, R.D., Anton, R.F., Jr., George, T.P., Greenfield, S.F., Kosten, T.R., *et al.* (2007). Treatment of patients with substance use disorders, second edition. Work Group on Substance Use Disorders, American Psychiatric Association. *American Journal of Psychiatry*, 164: 5–123. http://www.psychiatryonline.com/pracGuide/loadGuidelinePdf.aspx?file=SUD2ePG_04-28-06

Klein, T.W., Newton, C.A. & Friedman, H. (2001). Cannabinoids and the immune system. *Pain Research and Management*, 6: 95–101.

Klonoff-Cohen, H.S., Natarajan, L. & Chen, R.V. (2006). A prospective study of the effects of female and male marijuana use on in vitro fertilization (IVF) and gamete intrafallopian transfer (GIFT) outcomes. *American Journal of Obstetrics and Gynecology*, 194: 369–76.

Kolodny, R.C., Masters, W.H., Kolodner, R.M. & Toro, G. (1974). Depression of plasma testosterone levels after chronic intensive marihuana use. *New England Journal of Medicine*, 290: 872–4.

Korf, D. (2008). An open front door: The coffee shop phenomenon in the Netherlands. In: Rödner Sznitman, S., Olsson, B. & Room, R. (eds.) (2008). *A Cannabis Reader: Global Issues And Local Experiences*, vol. 1, pp. 140–54. Lisbon, European Monitoring Center on Drugs and Drug Abuse. http://www.emcdda.europa.eu/publications/monographs/cannabis

Korf, D. J. (2002). Dutch coffee shops and trends in cannabis use. *Addictive Behaviors, 27*(6): 851–66.

Korf, D., Brochu, S., Benschop, A.L. Harrison & P. Erickson (2008). 'Teen drug sellers – An international study of segregated drug markets and related violence' *Contemporary Drug Problems*, 35: 153–76.

Kouri, E.M. & Pope, H.G. (2000). Abstinence symptoms during withdrawal from chronic marijuana use. *Experimental and Clinical Psychopharmacology*, 8: 483–92.

Krajewski, K. (1999). How Flexible are the UN Drug Conventions? *The International Journal of Drug Policy*, 10(4): 329–38.

Ku, J. (2005a). The ICJ v. WTO: The EU's compliance with one treaty may violate another. *Opinio Juris weblog*, 19 May. http://lawofnations.blogspot.com/2005/05/icj-v-wto-eus-compliance-with-one.html

Ku, J. (2005b). Treaties as laws: A defense of the last in time rule for treaties and federal statutes. *Indiana Law Journal*, 80: 319–91. http://papers.ssrn.com/sol3/papers.cfm?abstract_id=597961

Kuijten, R.R., Bunin, G.R., Nass, C.C. & Meadows, A.T. (1992). Parental occupation and childhood astrocytoma – results of a case control study. *Cancer Research*, 52: 782–6.

Kumm, M. & Comella, V.F. (2004). *Altneuland: The EU Constitution in a Contextual Perspective*. New York: New York University School of Law, Jean Monnet Working Paper 5/04. http://www.jeanmonnetprogram.org/papers/04/040501-15.pdf

Lacey, M. (2009) In Mexico, ambivalence on a drug law. *New York Times*, 24 August. http://www.nytimes.com/2009/08/24/world/americas/24mexico.html?pagewanted=all

Lamarque, S., Taghzouti, K. & Simon, H. (2001). Chronic treatment with [Delta] 9-tetrahydrocannabinol enhances the locomotor response to amphetamine and heroin: implications for vulnerability to drug addiction. *Neuropharmacology*, 41: 118–29.

Lattimore, P., Broner, N. & Sherman, R. (2003). A comparison of prebooking and postbooking programs for mentally ill substance-using individuals with justice involvement. *Journal of Contemporary Criminal Justice*, 19: 30–64.

Laumon, B., Gadegbeku, B., Martin, J.L. & Biecheler, M.B. (2005). Cannabis intoxication and fatal road crashes in France: Population based case-control study. *BMJ*, 331: 1371.

Ledent, C., Valverde, O., Cossu, C., Petitet, F., Aubert, L.F., Beslot, F., *et al.* (1999). Unresponsiveness to cannabinoids and reduced addictive effects of opiates in CB1 receptor knockout mice. *Science*, 283: 401–04.

Leggett, T. (2008). A review of the world cannabis situation. *Bulletin on Narcotics* 58(1 & 2): 1–155 [issue dated 2006 but published 2008]. http://www.unodc.org/unodc/en/data-and-analysis/bulletin_2006-01-01_1.html

Leggett, T. & Pietschmann, T. (2008). Global cannabis cultivation and production. In: Rödner Sznitman, S., Olsson, B. & Room, R. (eds.) (2008). *A Cannabis Reader: Global Issues and Local Experiences*, vol. 1, pp. 187–212. Lisbon, European Monitoring Center on Drugs and Drug Abuse. http://www.emcdda.europa.eu/publications/monographs/cannabis

Legleye, S., Ben Lakhdar, C. & Spika, S. (2005). Two ways of estimating the Euro value of the illicit market for cannabis in France. *Drug and Alcohol Review*, 25(5): 466–72.

Leigh, L. (2007). The seamless web? Diversion from the criminal process and judicial review. *The Modern Law Review*, 70: 654–79.

Leinwand, M.A. (1971). The international law of treaties and United States legalization of marijuana. *Columbia Journal of Transnational Law,* 10: 413–41.

Lemmens, P. & Garretsen, H. (1998). Unstable pragmatism: Dutch drug policy under national and international pressure. *Addiction,* 93: 157–62.

Lenton, S. (2005a). Deterrence theory and the limitations of criminal penalties for cannabis use. In: T. Stockwell, P. Gruenewald, J. Toumbourou & W. Loxley (eds.), *Preventing Harmful Substance Use: The Evidence Base for Policy and Practice.* Chichester: John Wiley & Sons.

Lenton, S. (2005b). Evaluation of Western Australian Cannabis Infringement Notice Scheme – An overview. *Drug and Alcohol Review,* 24: 297–9.

Lenton, S. (2007). The WA Cannabis Infringement Notice Scheme: Reflections on the first 3 years. Invited plenary presentation at the Working Out What Works Symposium. Fremantle, 18–19 September 2007.

Lenton, S., Christie, P., Humeniuk, R., Brooks, A., Bennett, P. & Heale, P. (1999a). *Infringement versus conviction: The social impact of a minor cannabis offence under a civil penalties system and strict prohibition in two Australian states (monograph No. 36).* Canberra: Publications Productions Unit, Commonwealth Department of Health and Aged Care, National Drug Strategy.

Lenton, S., Ferrante, A. & Loh, N. (1996). Dope busts in the West: Minor cannabis offenses in the criminal justice system in Western Australia. *Drug and Alcohol Review,* 15: 335–41.

Lenton, S. & Heale, P. (2000). Arrest, court and social impacts of conviction for a minor cannabis offence under strict prohibition. *Contemporary Drug Problems,* 27: 805–33.

Lenton, S., Heale, P., Erickson, P., Single, E., Lang, E. & Hawks, D. (2000). *The Regulation of Cannabis Possession, Use and Supply: A Discussion Document Prepared for the Drugs and Crime Prevention Committee of the Parliament of Victoria.* NDRI Monograph No. 3. Perth: National Drug Research Institute, Curtin University of Technology.

Lenton, S., McDonald, D., Ali, R. & Moore, T. (1999b). Laws applying to minor cannabis offences in Australia and their evaluation. *International Journal of Drug Policy,* 10: 299–303.

Lessem, J.M., Hopfer, C.J., Haberstick, B.C., Timberlake, D., Ehringer, M.A., Smolen, A., et al. (2006). Relationship between adolescent marijuana use and young adult illicit drug use. *Behavior Genetics,* 36: 498–506.

Lichtman, A.H. & Martin, B.R. (2005). Cannabinoid tolerance and dependence. *Handbook of Experimental Pharmacology,* 168: 691–717.

Lichtman, A.H., Fisher, J. & Martin, B.R. (2001). Precipitated cannabinoid withdrawal is reversed by Delta(9)-tetrahydrocannabinol or clonidine. *Pharmacology, Biochemistry and Behavior,* 69: 181–8.

Lifrak, P.D., McKay, J.R., Rostain, A., Alterman, A.I. & Obrien, C.P. (1997). Relationship of perceived competencies, perceived social support, and gender to substance use in young adolescents. *Journal of the American Academy of Child and Adolescent Psychiatry,* 36: 933–40.

Llewellyn, C.D., Linklater, K., Bell, J., Johnson, N.W. & Warnakulasuriya, S. (2004). An analysis of risk factors for oral cancer in young people: A case-control study. *Oral Oncology,* 40: 304–13.

Loeber, R.T. & Yurgelun-Todd, D.A. (1999). Human neuroimaging of acute and chronic marijuana use: Implications for frontocerebellar dysfunction. *Human Psychopharmacology – Clinical and Experimental*, 14: 291–304.

Longo, M.C., Hunter, C.E., Lokan, R.J., White, J.M. & White, M.A. (2000). The prevalence of alcohol, cannabinoids, benzodiazepines and stimulants amongst injured drivers and their role in driver culpability. Part II: the relationship between drug prevalence and drug concentration, and driver culpability. *Accident Analysis and Prevention*, 32: 623–32.

Longshore, D., Evans, E., Urada, D., Teruya, C., Hardy, M., Hser, Y., *et al.* (2003). *Evaluation of the Substance Abuse and Crime Prevention Act 2002 Report.* Report Prepared for the Department of Alcohol and Drug Programs, California Health and Human Services Agency. Los Angeles: University of California Los Angeles UCLA.

Loxley, W., Gray, D., Wilkinson, C., Chikritzhs, T., Midford, R. & Moore, D. (2005). Alcohol policy and harm reduction in Australia. *Drug and Alcohol Review*, 24(5), 559–68.

Lubman, D. I., Yucel, M. & Hall, W. D. (2007). Substance use and the adolescent brain: A toxic combination? *J Psychopharmacol, 21*(8): 792–4.

Lucas, P. (2008). Regulating compassion: An overview of Canada's federal medical cannabis policy and practice. *Harm Reduction Journal*, 5: 1–13.

Lundqvist, T., Jonsson, S. & Warkentin, S. (2001). Frontal lobe dysfunction in long-term cannabis users. *Neurotoxicology and Teratology*, 23: 437–43.

Lyketsos, C.G., Garrett, E., Liang, K.Y. & Anthony, J.C. (1999). Cannabis use and cognitive decline in persons under 65 years of age. *American Journal of Epidemiology*, 149: 794–800.

Lynskey, M.T. (2002). An alternative model is feasible, but the gateway hypothesis has not been invalidated: Comments on Morral *et al. Addiction*, 97: 1505–07.

Lynskey, M.T. & Hall, W.D. (2000). The effects of adolescent cannabis use on educational attainment: A review. *Addiction*, 96: 433–43.

Lynskey, M.T., Heath, A.C., Bucholz, K.K. & Slutske, W.S. (2003). Escalation of drug use in early-onset cannabis users vs co-twin controls. *JAMA*, 289: 427–33.

Lynskey, M.T., Vink, J.M. & Boomsma, D.I. (2006). Early onset cannabis use and progression to other drug use in a sample of Dutch twins. *Behavior Genetics*, 36: 195–200.

Lynskey, M.T., White, V., Hill, D., Letcher, T. & Hall, W.D. (1999). Prevalence of illicit drug use among youth: Results from the Australian school students' alcohol and drugs survey. *Australian and New Zealand Journal of Public Health*, 23: 519–24.

MacCoun, R. & Reuter, P. (1997). Interpreting Dutch cannabis policy: Reasoning by analogy in the legalisation debate. *Science*, 278(3): 47–52.

MacCoun, R. & Reuter, P. (2001a). Comparative cannabis use data – Authors reply. *Br J Psychiatry*, 179(2): 175–7.

MacCoun, R. & Reuter, P. (2001b). Evaluating alternative cannabis regimes. *British Journal of Psychiatry*, 178: 123–8.

Macintosh, A. (2006). *Drug Law Reform: Beyond Prohibition*. Report Discussion Paper Number 83. Canberra: The Australian Institute. https://www.tai.org.au/file. php?file=DP83.pdf

Macleod, J., Oakes, R., Copello, A., Crome, I., Egger, M., Hickman, M., *et al.* (2004). Psychological and social sequelae of cannabis and other illicit drug use by young people: a systematic review of longitudinal, general population studies. *Lancet*, 363: 1579–88.

MacPhee, D. (1999). Effects of marijuana on cell nuclei: A review of the literature relating to the genotoxicity of cannabis. In: Kalant, H., Corrigall, W., Hall, W.D. & Smart, R. (eds.), *The Health Effects of Cannabis*. Toronto: Centre for Addiction and Mental Health, pp. 435–458.

Maldonado, R. (2002). Study of cannabinoid dependence in animals. *Pharmacology and Therapeutics*, 95: 153–64.

Manfredi, C. & Maioni, A. (2002). Courts and health policy: Judicial policy making and publicly funded health care in Canada. *Journal of Health Politics, Policy and Law*, 27: 213–40.

Mannisto, P. & Kaakkola, S. (2006). Catechol-O-methyltransferase (COMT): Biochemistry, molecular biology, pharmacology, and clinical efficacy of the new selective COMT inhibitors. *Pharmacological Reviews*, 51: 593–628.

Manzanares, J., Corchero, J., Romero, J., Fernandez-Ruiz, J.J., Ramos, J.A. & Fuentes, J.A. (1999). Pharmacological and biochemical interactions between opioids and cannabinoids. *Trends in Pharmacological Sciences*, 20: 287–94.

Marijuana Policy Project (2007). *State-by-State Medical Marijuana Laws: How to Remove the Threat of Arrest*. Capitol Hill, Washington DC: Marijuana Policy Project.

Marselos, M. & Karamanakos, P. (1999). Mutagenicity, developmental toxicity and carcinogeneity of cannabis. *Addiction Biology*, 4: 5–12.

May, T. (2007). personal communication, 11/10/2007.

May, T., Duffy, M., Warburton, H. & Hough, M. (2007). *Policing cannabis as a Class C drug: an arresting change?* York, UK: Joseph Rowntree Foundation.

McCoy, Alfred W. (1991). *The Politics of Heroin: CIA Complicity in the Global Drug Trade.* Brooklyn, NY: Lawrence Hill Books.

McDonald, D., Moore, R., Norberry, J., Wardlaw, G. & Ballenden, N. (1994). *Legislative Options for Cannabis in Australia*. Canberra: Australian Government Publishing Service.

McGee, R. & Feehan, M. (1993). Cannabis use among New Zealand adolescents. *New Zealand Medical Journal*, 106: 345.

McGee, R., Williams, S., Poulton, R. & Moffitt, T. (2000). A longitudinal study of cannabis use and mental health from adolescence to early adulthood. *Addiction*, 95: 491–503.

McGeorge, J. & Aitken, C. K. (1997). Effects of cannabis decriminalization in the Australian capital territory on university students' patterns of use. *Journal of Drug Issues,* 27(4): 785–93.

McLaren, J., Swift, W., Dillon, P. & Allsop, S. (2008). Cannabis potency and contamination: A review of the literature. *Addiction*, 103: 1100–109.

McRae, A.L., Budney, A.J. & Brady, K.T. (2003). Treatment of marijuana dependence: A review of the literature. *Journal of Substance Abuse Treatment*, 24: 369–376.

Mehra, R., Moore, B.A., Crothers, K., Tetrault, J. & Fiellin, D.A. (2006). The association between marijuana smoking and lung cancer: a systematic review. *Archives of Internal Medicine*, 166: 1359–67.

Mellinger, G.D., Somers, R.H., Davidson, S.T. & Manheimer, S.H. (1976). The amotivational syndrome and the college student. *Annals of the New York Academy of Sciences*, 282: 37–55.

Mendelson, J.H. & Mello, N.K. (1984). Effects of marijuana on neuroendocrine hormones in human males and females. In Braude, M. & Ludford, J.P. (eds.), *Marijuana Effects on the Endocrine and Reproductive Systems*. Rockville, MD: National Institute on Drug Abuse.

Mendelson, J.H., Kuehnle, J., Ellingboe, J. & Babor, T.F. (1974). Plasma testosterone levels before, during and after chronic marihuana smoking. *New England Journal of Medicine*, 291: 1051–5.

Miller, J. & Lang, A. (2007). *ASSAD Drug Report 2005*. Canberra: TNS Social Research.

Mills, J.H. (2003). *Cannabis Britannica: Empire, Trade, and Prohibition 1800–1928*. New York: Oxford University Press.

Miron, J. O. (2002). *The Effect of Marijuana Decriminalization on the Budgets of Massachusetts Governments, With a Discussion of Decriminalization's Effect on Marijuana Use*. Massachusettes: Drug Policy Forum of Massachusetts.

Mittleman, M.A., Lewis, R.A., Maclure, M., Sherwood, J.B. & Muller, J.E. (2001). Triggering myocardial infarction by marijuana. *Circulation*, 103: 2805–09.

Model, K.E. (1993). The effect of marijuana decriminalisation on hospital emergency room drug episodes: 1975–1978. *Journal of the American Statistical Association*, 88(423): 737–47.

Moir, D., Rickert, W.S., Levasseur, G., Larose, Y., Maertens, R., White, P., *et al*. (2008). A comparison of mainstream and sidestream marijuana and tobacco cigarette smoke produced under two machine smoking conditions. *Chemical Research in Toxicology*, 21: 494–502.

Monshouwer, K., Smit, F., Graaf, R.D., Os, J.V. & Vollebergh, W. (2005). First cannabis use: Does onset shift to younger ages? Findings from 1988 to 2003 from the Dutch National School Survey on Substance Use. *Addiction*, 100: 963–70.

Montanari, L., Taylor, C. & Griffiths, P. (2008). Cannabis users in drug treatment in Europe: an analysis from treatment demand data. In: Rödner Sznitman, S., Olsson, B. & Room, R. (eds.) (2008), *A cannabis reader: global issues and local experiences*, vol. 2, pp. 263–276. Lisbon: European Monitoring Center on Drugs and Drug Abuse. http://www.emcdda.europa.eu/publications/monographs/cannabis

Moore, T.H., Zammit, S., Lingford-Hughes, A., Barnes, T.R., Jones, P.B., Burke, M., *et al*. (2007). Cannabis use and risk of psychotic or affective mental health outcomes: A systematic review. *Lancet*, 370: 319–28.

Morahan, P.S., Klykken, P.C., Smith, S.H., Harris, L.S. & Munson, A.E. (1979). Effects of cannabinoids on host resistance to Listeria monocytogenes and herpes simplex virus. *Infection and Immunity*, 23: 670–4.

Moravek, J. (2008). Problem drug use, marijuana, and European projects: How epidemiology helped Czech drug reformers. *Central European Journal of Public Policy*, 2(2), 26–39. http://www.cejpp.eu/index.php/volume-2-number-2-december-2008/view-category.html

Morgan, C.J. & Curran, H.V. (2008). Effects of cannabidiol on schizophrenia-like symptoms in people who use cannabis. *British Journal of Psychiatry*, 192: 306–07.

Morral, A.R., McCaffrey, D.F. & Paddock, S.M. (2002). Reassessing the marijuana gateway effect. *Addiction*, 97: 1493–504.

Mukamal, K.J., Maclure, M., Muller, J.E. & Mittleman, M.A. (2008). An exploratory prospective study of marijuana use and mortality following acute myocardial infarction. *American Heart Journal*, 155: 465–70.

Mura, P., Kintz, P., Ludes, B., Gaulier, J.M., Marquet, P., Martin-Dupont, S., *et al.* (2003). Comparison of the prevalence of alcohol, cannabis and other drugs between 900 injured drivers and 900 control subjects: results of a French collaborative study. *Forensic Science International*, 133: 79–85.

Murphy, L. (1999). Cannabis effects on endocrine and reproductive function. In: Kalant, H., Corrigall, W., Hall, W.D. & Smart, R. (eds.), *The Health Effects of Cannabis*. Toronto: Centre for Addiction and Mental Health, pp. 375–400.

Murray, R.M., Morrison, P.D., Henquet, C. & Di Forti, M. (2007). Cannabis, the mind and society: the hash realities. *Nature Reviews Neuroscience*, 8: 885–895.

Nahas, G.G. (1990). *Keep off the Grass*. Middlebury, VT: Paul Eriksson.

National Association of Drug Court Professionals (NADCP) (1999). *Facts on Drug Courts*. Alexandria, VA: NADCP. http://www.nadcp.org/whatis/

National Drug Intelligence Center (2008). *National Drug Threat Assessment 2008*. Johnstown, Pennsylvania: NDIC.

National Organization for the Reform of Marijuana Laws (NORML) (2008). NORML *Working to Reform Marijuana Laws*. http://norml.org/

Neglia, J., Buckley, J. & Robinson, L. (1991). Maternal marijuana and leukemia in offspring. In: Nahas, G.G. & Latour, C. (eds.), *Physiopathology of Illicit Drugs: Cannabis, Cocaine, Opiates*. Oxford: Pergamon.

Neill, M., Christie, P. & Cormack, S. (1991). *Trends in Alcohol and Other Drug Use By South Australian School Children 1986–1989*. Adelaide: Drug and Alcohol Services Council South Australia.

Newcomb, M.D. & Bentler, P.M. (1988). *Consequences of Adolescent Drug Use: Impact on the Lives of Young Adults*. Thousand Oaks, CA: Sage.

Nicholas, S., Kershaw, C. & Walker, A. (eds.). (2007). *Home Office Statistical Bulletin: Crime in England and Wales 2006/07* (4th edn). London: Home Office.

Niesink, R., Rigter, S. & Hoek, J. (2005). *THC-concentraties in wiet, nederwiet en hasj in Nederlandse coffeeshops (2004–2005)* Utrecht, Netherlands: Trimbos Institute.

Nordt, C. & Stohler, R. (2006). Incidence of heroin use in Zurich, Swizerland; a treatment case register analysis. *The Lancet*, 367: 1830–1834.

Nutt, D., King, L.A., Saulsbury, W. & Blakemore, C. (2007). Development of a rational scale to assess the harm of drugs of potential misuse. *Lancet*, 369: 1047–53.

NZZ Online (2008). Cannabis-Konsum soll nicht straffrei werden. http://www.nzz.ch/nachrichten/schweiz/auch_staenderat_spricht_sich_gegen_hanf-initiative_aus_1.687299.html

Office of National Drug Control Policy (2001). *What America's Users Spend on Illicit Drugs: 1988–2001*. Washington, D.C.: ONDCP.

ONDCP (2007). *Study Finds Highest Levels of THC in U.S. Marijuana to Date [release]*. Washington, DC: Office of National Drug Control Policy. Available at: http://www.whitehousedrugpolicy.gov/news/press07/042507_2.html.

Office of National Drug Control Policy (2008). *The Price and Purity of Illicit Drugs 1981–2007*. http://www.whitehousedrugpolicy.gov/publications/price_purity/price_purity07.pdf [accessed April 11, 2009]

Pacula, R.L., Chriqui, J.F. & King, J. (2003). *Decriminalization in the United States: What does it mean?* NBER Working Paper, No. 9690. New York: NBER.

Pacula, R., Chriqui, J., Reichmann, D. & Terry-McElrath, Y. (2002). State Medical Marijuana Laws: Understanding the Laws and their Limitations. *Journal of Public Health Policy*, 23: 413–39.

Pacula, R., MacCoun, R., Reuter, P., Chriqui, J., Kilmer, B., Harris, K., Paoli, L. & Schafer, C. (2005). What does it mean to decriminalize marijuana? A cross-national empirical examination. *Advances in Health Economics and Health Services Research*, 16: 347–69.

Pakes, F. (2004). The politics of discontent: The emergence of a new criminal justice discourse in the Netherlands. *The Howard Journal*, 43: 284–98.

Paoli, L., Greenfield, V. & Reuter, P. (in press). *Can Global Heroin Supply be Cut?* Oxford: Oxford University Press.

Passey, M., Flaherty, B. & Didcott, P. (2006). The Magistrates Early Referral Into Treatment (MERIT) Pilot Program: A descriptive analysis of a court diversion program in rural Australia. *Journal of Psychoactive Drugs*, 38: 521–9.

Patton, G.C., Coffey, C., Carlin, J.B., Degenhardt, L., Lynskey, M.T. & Hall, W.D. (2002). Cannabis use and mental health in young people: Cohort study. *British Medical Journal*, 325: 1195–8.

Patton, G.C., Harris, J.B., Schwartz, M. & Bowes, G. (1997). Adolescent suicidal behaviors: A population-based study of risk. *Psychological Medicine*, 27: 715–24.

Pauwelyn, J. (2003). *Conflict of Norms in Public International Law: How WTO Law Relates to Other Rules of International Law*. Cambridge, etc.: Cambridge University Press.

Pearson, G. (2007). The policing of cannabis in the United Kingdom. *Addiction*, 102: 1175–7.

Perez-Gomez, A. (2005). *Drug Consumption in Colombia*, 1992–2003. Unpublished paper.

Perkonigg, A., Goodwin, R.D., Fiedler, A., Behrendt, S., Beesdo, K., Lieb, R. & Wittchen H.U. (2008). The natural course of cannabis use, abuse and dependence during the first decades of life. *Addiction*, 103(3): 439–49.

Pertwee, R.G. (2008). The diverse CB1 and CB2 receptor pharmacology of three plant cannabinoids: Delta9-tetrahydrocannabinol, cannabidiol and delta9-tetrahydrocannabivarin. *British Journal of Pharmacology*, 153: 199–215.

Pijlman, F.T., Rigter, S.M., Hoek, J., Goldschmidt, H.M. & Niesink, R.J. (2005). Strong increase in total delta-THC in cannabis preparations sold in Dutch coffee shops. *Addiction Biology*, 10: 171–80.

Polak, F. (1998). The boundaries of decriminalisation: Coffee shops and the backdoor problem. Paper presented at the symposium, Regulating cannabis: Options for control in the 21st century, London, 5 September.

Pope, H.G., Gruber, A.J. & Yurgelun-Todd, D. (1995). The residual neuropsychological effects of cannabis: The current status of research. *Drug and Alcohol Dependence*, 38: 25–34.

Pope, H.G., Gruber, A.J., Hudson, J.I., Huestis, M.A. & Yurgelun-Todd, D. (2001). Neuropsychological performance in long-term cannabis users. *Archives of General Psychiatry*, 58: 909–15.

Pope, H.G., Gruber, A.J., Hudson, J.I., Huestis, M.A. & Yurgelun-Todd, D. (2002). Cognitive measures in long-term cannabis users. *Journal of Clinical Pharmacology*, 42: 41S–47S.

Porrino, L.J., Whitlow, C.T., Lamborn, C., Laurienti, P.J. & Livengood, L.B. (2004). Impaired performance on a decision-making task by heavy marijuana users: An fMRI study. *Symposium on the Cannabinoids.* Burlington, VT: International Cannabinoid Research Society.

Potter, D.J., Clark, P. & Brown, M.B. (2008). Potency of delta 9-THC and other cannabinoids in cannabis in England in 2005: implications for psychoactivity and pharmacology. *Journal of Forensic Sciences,* 53: 90–4.

Priori, J., Swensen, G., Migro, J., Tomassini, R., Marshall, A. & Lenton, S. (2002). *Implementation of a Scheme of Prohibition with Civil Penalties for the Personal Use of Cannabis and Other Matters – Report of the Working Party on Drug Law Reform to the Minister for Health.* Perth: Drug and Alcohol Office, Health Department of Western Australia.

Pudney, S. (2004). Keeping off the grass? An econometric model of cannabis consumption in Britain. *Journal of Applied Econometrics,* 19: 435–53.

Pudney, S., Badillo, C. Bryan, M., Burton, J., Conti, G. & Iacovou, M. (2006). Estimating the size of the UK illicit drug market. In: Singleton, N., Murray, R. & Tinsley, L. (eds.), *Measuring Different Aspects of Problem Use: Methodological Developments.* Home Office online report 16/2006, 46–120, available at: http://www.homeoffice.gov.uk

Quickfall, J. & Crockford, D. (2006). Brain neuroimaging in cannabis use: A review. *Journal of Neuropsychiatry and Clinical Neurosciences,* 18: 318–32.

Ramaekers, J.G., Berghaus, G., van Laar, M. & Drummer, O.H. (2004). Dose related risk of motor vehicle crashes after cannabis use. *Drug and Alcohol Dependence,* 73: 109–19.

Rehm, J., Gnam, W., Popova, S., Baliunas, D., Brochu, S., Fischer, B., *et al.* (2007). The costs of alcohol, illegal drugs, and tobacco in Canada, 2002. *Journal of Studies on Alcohol and Drugs,* 68: 886–895.

Reinarman, C., Cohen, P.D.A. & Kaal, H.L. (2004). The limited relevance of drug policy: Cannabis in Amsterdam and in San Francisco. *American Journal of Public Health,* 94(5): 836–42.

Reis, L., Eisner, M., Kosary, C., Hankey, B., Miller, B., Clegg, L., *et al.* (eds.) (2000). *SEER Cancer Statistics Review, 1973–1997.* Bethesda, MD: National Cancer Institute.

Resnick, M.D., Bearman, P.S., Blum, R.W., Bauman, K.E., Harris, K.M., Jones, J., *et al.* (1997). Protecting adolescents from harm: Findings from the National Longitudinal Study on Adolescent Health. *JAMA,* 278: 823–32.

Reuter, P., Hirschfield, P. & Davies, K. (2001). *Assessing the Crackdown on Marijuana in Maryland.* unpublished paper, U. of Maryland. http://www.drugpolicy.org/docUploads/md_mj_crackdown.pdf

Rey, J.M., Sawyer, M.G., Raphael, B., Patton, G.C. & Lynskey, M.T. (2002). Mental health of teenagers who use cannabis: Results of an Australian survey. *British Journal of Psychiatry,* 180: 216–21.

Robbe, H.W.J. (1994). *Influence of Marijuana on Driving.* Maastricht: Institute for Human Psychopharmacology, University of Limberg.

Roberts, J. & Cole, D. (1999). *Making Sense of Sentencing.* Toronto: University of Toronto Press.

Robinson, L., Buckley, J., Daigle, A., Wells, R., Benjamin, D., Arthur, D., *et al.* (1989). Maternal drug use and the risk of childhood nonlymphoblastic leukemia among offspring: An epidemiologic investigation implicating marijuana. *Cancer*, 63: 1904–1911.

Rödner Sznitman, S., Olsson, B. & Room, R. (eds.) (2008). *A Cannabis Reader: Global Issues and Local Experiences.* Lisbon, European Monitoring Center on Drugs and Drug Abuse. http://www.emcdda.europa.eu/publications/monographs/cannabis

Roffman, R.A. & Stephens, R.S. (2006). *Cannabis Dependence: Its Nature, Consequences and Treatment.* Cambridge; New York: Cambridge University Press.

Room, R. (1999). The rhetoric of international drug control. *Substance Use and Misuse,* 34: 1689–1707.

Room, R. (2005). Trends and issues in the international drug control system: Vienna 2003. *Journal of Psychoactive Drugs,* 37(4): 373–83.

Room, R. (2006). International control of alcohol: alternative paths forward. *Drug and Alcohol Review,* 25(6): 581–95.

Room, R. & Paglia, A. (1999). The international drug control system in the post-Cold War era: Managing markets or fighting a war? *Drug and Alcohol Review,* 18(3): 305–15.

Roques, B., chair (1999). *La Dangerosité de Drogues: Rapport au Secrétariat d'État à la Santé* [The Dangerousness of Drugs: Report to the State Secretariat for Health]. Paris: La Documentation française-Odile Jacob.

Rosenblatt, K.A., Daling, J.R., Chen, C., Sherman, K.J. & Schwartz, S.M. (2004). Marijuana use and risk of oral squamous cell carcinoma. *Cancer Research*, 64: 4049–54.

Roth, M.D., Baldwin, G.C. & Tashkin, D.P. (2002). Effects of delta-9-tetrahydrocannabinol on human immune function and host defense. *Chemistry and Physics of Lipids*, 121: 229–39.

Rush, B. & Urbanosk, K. (2007). Estimating the demand for treatment for cannabis-related problems in Canada. *International Journal of Mental Health and Addiction*, 5(3): 181–6.

SAMHSA (2004). *Treatment Episode Data Set (TEDS): Highlights, 2002. National Admissions to Substance Abuse Treatment Services.* Rockville, MD: Office of Applied Studies, Substance and Mental Health Services Administration.

SAMHSA (2006). *Results from the 2005 National Survey on Drug Use and Health: Detailed Tables. Prevalence Estimates, Standard Errors, P Values. Section 1.* Rockville, MD: Substance Abuse and Mental Health Administration, Office of Applied Studies. Available at: http://www.oas.samhsa.gov.

Samuels, D. (2008). Dr. Kush: How medical marijuana is transforming the pot industry. *New Yorker*, July 28. http://www.newyorker.com/reporting/2008/07/28/080728fa_fact_samuels

Sarre, R., Sutton, A. & Pulsford, T. (1989). *Cannabis – The Expiation Notice Approach. (Report Series C, No. 4, June)* Adelaide: South Australian Attorney General's Department.

Saveland, W. & Bray, D.F. (1981). Trends in cannabis use among American states with different and changing legal regimes, 1972–77. *Contemporary Drug Problems*, 10: 335–61.

Schafer, C. & Paoli, L. (2006). *Drogen und Strafverfolgung: Die Anwendung des § 31 a BtMG und anderer Opportunitätsvorschriften auf Drogenkonsumentendelikte.* Freiburg: Max Planck Institut für Ausländisches und Internationales Strafrecht.

Schlosser, E. (1994). Reefer Madness. *The Atlantic Monthly*, 274: 45–58.

Schmid, H. (2001). Cannabis use in Switzerland: The role of attribution of drug use to friends, urbanization and repression. *Swiss Journal of Psychology*, 60(2): 99–107.

Schweizer Bundesrat (2001). *Botschaft uber die Anderung des Betaubungsmittelgesetzes.* Berne: Bundesrat.

Schweizerische Eidgenossenschaft (2007). *Polizeiliche Kriminalstatistik.* Berne: Bundesamt für Statistik.

Selley, D.A., Lichtman, A.H. & Martin, B.R. (2003). Integration of molecular and behavioral approaches to evaluate cannabinoid dependence. In Maldonado, R. (ed.), *Molecular Biology of Drug Addiction.* Totowa, NJ: Humana Press, pp. 199–220.

Senate Special Committee on Illegal Drugs (2002). *Cannabis: Our Position for a Canadian Public Policy.* Ottawa: Canadian Parliament, Senate.

Sharma, A. (2007). Starting the day with the cup that kicks. *Hindustan Times*, 4 November. http://www.hindustantimes.com/StoryPage/StoryPage.aspx?id=8d0650c1-e9d9-4f7e-a683-6b3cc8bdd778

Shepard, E. & Blackley, P. (2007). The impact of marijuana law enforcement in an economic model of crime. *Journal of Drug Issues*, 37: 403–24.

Sherman, L., Gottfredson, D., MacKenzie, D., Eck, J., Reuter, P. & Bushway, S. (1998). *Preventing Crime: What Works, What Doesn't, What's Promising – A Report to the United States Congress.* College Park: Department of Criminology and Criminal Justice, University of Maryland.

Sibbald, B. (2002). Medical Marijuana Program 'a sham': Lawyer. *Canadian Medical Association Journal*, 167: 1153.

Sidney, S. (2002). Cardiovascular consequences of marijuana use. *Journal of Clinical Pharmacology*, 42: 64S–70S.

Sidney, S., Beck, J.E., Tekawa, I.S., Quesenberry, C.P. & Friedman, G.D. (1997a). Marijuana use and mortality. *American Journal of Public Health*, 87: 585–90.

Sidney, S., Quesenberry, C.P., Jr., Friedman, G.D. & Tekawa, I.S. (1997b). Marijuana use and cancer incidence (California, United States). *Cancer Causes and Control*, 8: 722–8.

Silver, W. (2007). Canadian Crime Statistics, 2006. *Juristat.* Vol. 27, no.5. Catalogue 85-002-XIE. Ottawa: Statistics Canada. http://www.statcan.ca/english/freepub/85-002-XIE/85-002-XIE2007005.pdf

Single, E. (1989). The impact of marijuana decriminalisation: An update. *Journal of Public Health Policy*, 10(Winter): 456–66.

Slaughter, J. (1988). Marijuana Prohibition in the United States: History and analysis of a failed policy. *Columbia Journal of Law and Social Problems*, 21: 417–75.

Smiley, A. (1999). Marijuana: on road and driving simulator studies. In: Kalant, H., Corrigall, W., Hall, W.D. & Smart, R. (eds.), *The Health Effects of Cannabis.* Toronto: Centre for Addiction and Mental Health, pp. 171–91.

Smit, F., Bolier, L. & Cuijpers, P. (2004). Cannabis use and the later risk of schozophrenia: A review. *Addiction*, 99: 422–31.

Smith, A.M., Fried, P.A., Hogan, M.J. & Cameron, I. (2004). Effects of prenatal marijuana on response inhibition: An fMRI study of young adults. *Neurotoxicology and Teratology*, 26: 533–42.

Smith, D. & Visher, C. (1981). Street-level justice: Situational determinants of police arrest decisions. *Social Problems*, 29: 167–77.

Smith, M.A., Gloekler, Reis, L., Gurney, J. & Ross, J. (2000). Leukemia. In: Reis, L., Eisner, M., Kosary, C., Hankey, B., Miller, B., Clegg, L., *et al.* (eds.), *SEER Cancer Statistics Review, 1973–1997*. Bethesda, MD: National Cancer Institute, pp. 17–34.

Solivetti, L.M. (2001). *Drug Use Criminalization v. Decriminalization: An Analysis in the Light of the Italian Experience*. Bern: Swiss Federal Office of Public Health.

Solowij, N. (1998). *Cannabis and Cognitive Functioning*. Cambridge, UK: Cambridge University Press.

Solowij, N. (1999). Long-term effects of cannabis on the central nervous system. I. Brain function and neurotoxicity. II. Cognitive functioning. In Kalant, H., Corrigal, W., Hall, W. & Smart, R. (eds.), *The Health Effects of Cannabis*. Toronto: Centre for Addiction and Mental Health, pp. 195–265.

Solowij, N. (2002). Cannabis and cognitive functioning. In: Onaivi, E.S. (ed.), *Biology of Marijuana: From Gene to Behaviour*. London: Taylor & Francis.

Solowij, N., Respondek, C. & Ward, P. (2004). Functional magnetic resonance imaging indices of memory function in long-term cannabis users. *Symposium on the Cannabinoids*. Burlington, VT: International Cannabinoid Research Society.

Solowij, N., Stephens, R.S., Roffman, R.A., Babor, T., Kadden, R., Miller, M., *et al.* (2002). Cognitive functioning of long-term heavy cannabis users seeking treatment. *JAMA*, 287: 1123–31.

Sourcebook of Criminal Justice Statistcs (2007). http://www.albany.edu/sourcebook/toc.html

Spagnolo, J. (2009). Premier Colin Barnett's 2009 war on drugs. *PerthNow*, Jan 3. http://www.news.com.au/perthnow/story/0,,24868863-2761,00.html

Special Committee on Non-Medical Use of Drugs (2002). *Policy for the New Millenium: Working Together to Redefine Canada's Drug Strategy*. Ottawa: House of Commons.

Spivack, D. (2004). *A Fourth International Convention for Drug Policy: Promoting Public Health Policies*. Paris: The Senlis Council. http://www.senliscouncil.net/modules/publications/007_publication

Spooner, C. (2001). An overview of diversion strategies for Australian drug-related offenders. *Drug and Alcohol Review*, 20: 281–94.

Statistics Canada (2007). Cases in adults criminal court by type of sentences; total convicted cases, prison, conditional sentence, probation, by province and Yukon Territory. Report Table 252-0017 Catalogue no. 85-002-X. Ottawa: CANISM.

Stinson, F.S., Ruan, W.J., Pickering, R. & Grant, B.F. (2006). Cannabis use disorders in the USA: Prevalence, correlates and co-morbidity. *Psychological Medicine*, 36: 1447–60.

Strategy Unit (2005). *Strategy Unit Drugs Report, May 2003*. London: Prime Minister's Strategy Unit. Available at: http://www.strategy.gov.uk/work_areas/drugs/index.asp (Full report at http://image.guardian.co.uk/sys-files/Guardian/documents/2005/07/05/Report.pdf).

Stuart, R. B., Guire, K. & Krell, M. (1976). Penalty for the possession of marijuana: An analysis of some of its concomitants. *Contemporary Drug Problems, 5*: 553.

Substance Abuse and Mental Health Services Administration (2007). Office of Applied Studies. *Treatment Episode Data Set (TEDS) Highlights – 2006 National Admissions to Substance Abuse Treatment Services*. OAS Series #S-40, DHHS Publication No. (SMA) 08-4313, Rockville, MD http://www.oas.samhsa.gov/teds2k6highlights/Tbl4.htm [accessed September 1, 2008]

Sutton, A. & McMillan, E. (2000). Criminal justice perspectives on South Australia's Cannabis Expiation Notice procedures. *Drug and Alcohol Review*, 19(3): 281–6.

Swaine, E.T. (2006). Reserving. *Yale Journal of International Law*, 31: 307–66. http://www.yale.edu/yjil/PDFs/vol_31/Swaine.pdf

Swift, W., Hall, W.D. & Teesson, M. (2001). Cannabis use and dependence among Australian adults: Results from the National Survey of Mental Health and Well-being. *Addiction*, 96: 737–48.

Tanda, G., Pontieri, F.E. & Di Chiara, G. (1997). Cannabinoid and heroin activation of mesolimbic dopamine transmission by a common mu1 opioid receptor mechanism. *Science*, 276: 2048–50.

Tanner, J., Davies, S. & O'Grady, B. (1999). Whatever happened to yesterday's rebels? Longitudinal effects of youth delinquency on education and employment. *Social Problems*, 46: 250–274.

Tashkin, D.P. (1999). Effects of cannabis on the respiratory system. In: Kalant, H., Corrigall, W., Hall, W.D. & Smart, R. (eds.), *The Health Effects of Cannabis*. Toronto: Centre for Addiction and Mental Health.

Tashkin, D.P. (2005). Smoked marijuana as a cause of lung injury. *Monaldi Archives for Chest Disease*, 63: 93–100.

Tashkin, D.P., Baldwin, G.C., Sarafian, T., Dubinett, S. & Roth, M.D. (2002). Respiratory and immunologic consequences of marijuana smoking. *Journal of Clinical Pharmacology*, 42: 71S–81S.

Taxman, F. & Bouffard, J. (2002). Treatment inside the drug treatment court: The who, what, where, and how of treatment services. *Substance Use & Misuse*, 37: 1665–88.

Taylor, D.R., Fergusson, D.M., Milne, B.J., Horwood, L.J., Moffitt, T.E., Sears, M.R., *et al.* (2002). A longitudinal study of the effects of tobacco and cannabis exposure on lung function in young adults. *Addiction*, 97: 1055–61.

Taylor, D.R., Poulton, R., Moffitt, T., Ramankutty, P. & Sears, M. (2000). The respiratory effects of cannabis dependence in young adults. *Addiction*, 95: 1669–77.

Tennes, K., Aritable, N., Blackard, C., Boyles, C., Hasoun, B., Holmes, L., *et al.* (1985). Marihuana: Prenatal and postnatal exposure in the human. In: Pinkert, T. (ed.), *Current Research on the Consequences of Maternal Drug Abuse*. Rockville, MD: U. S. Department of Health and Human Services, pp. 48–60.

Tetrault, J.M., Crothers, K., Moore, B.A., Mehra, R., Concato, J. & Fiellin, D.A. (2007). Effects of marijuana smoking on pulmonary function and respiratory complications: a systematic review. *Archives of Internal Medicine*, 167: 221–8.

Theis, C. F. & Register, C. A. (1993). Decriminalisation of marijuana and the demand for alcohol, marijuana and cocaine. *The Social Science Journal*, 30(4): 385–9.

True, W.R., Heath, A.C., Scherrer, J.F., Xian, H., Lin, N., Eisen, S.A., *et al.* (1999). Interrelationship of genetic and environmental influences on conduct disorder and alcohol and marijuana dependence symptoms. *American Journal of Medical Genetics*, 88: 391–7.

Turner, S., Longshore, D., Wenzel, S., Deschenes, E., Greenwood, P., Fain, T., *et al.* (2002). A decade of drug treatment court research. *Substance Use & Misuse*, 37: 1489–1527.

Uitermark, J. (2004) The origins and future of the Dutch approach towards drugs. *Journal of Drug Issues* 34: 511–532.

UK Drug Policy Commission (2008). *Submission to the ACMD Cannabis Classification Review 2008.* London: UK Drug Policy Commission.

UKCIA (2000). *Major Political Research Studies.* Norwich: UK Cannabis Internet Activists. http://www.ukcia.org/politics/studies.html

Ulrich, T. (2002). Pretrial diversion in the federal court system. *Federal Probation*, 66: 30–7.

UN (2005a). *Vienna Convention on the Law of Treaties, 1969.* New York: United Nations. http://untreaty.un.org/ilc/texts/instruments/english/conventions/1_1_1969.pdf

UN (2005b). *Vienna Convention on the Law of Treaties between States and International Organizations or between International Organizations, 1986.* New York: United Nations. http://untreaty.un.org/ilc/texts/instruments/english/conventions/1_2_1986.pdf

UN (2007a). *Single Convention on Narcotic Drugs, 1961, as Amended by the 1972 Protocol Amending the Single Convention on Narcotic Drugs, 1961.* Vienna: International Narcotics Control Board. http://www.incb.org/pdf/e/conv/convention_1961_en.pdf

UN (2007b). *United Nations Convention against the Illicit Traffic in Narcotic Drugs and Psychotropic Substances, 1988.* Vienna: International Narcotics Control Board. http://www.incb.org/pdf/e/conv/convention_1988_en.pdf

UNESCO (2005). *International Convention against Doping in Sport 2005.* Paris: United Nations Educational, Scientific and Cultural Organization. http://portal.unesco.org/en/ev.php-URL_ID=31037&URL_DO=DO_TOPIC&URL_SECTION=201.html

UNIS (2008). *Marijuana vending machines in Los Angeles are contrary to international drug control treaties, says INCB.* Vienna: United Nations Information Service, UNIS/NAR/1023, 8 Feb. http://www.unis.unvienna.org/unis/pressrels/2008/unisnar1023.html

UNODC (2000). *World Drug Report 2000.* Oxford: Oxford University Press. http://www.unodc.org/unodc/en/data-and-analysis/WDR-2000.html

UNODC (2005). *World Drug Report 2005.* New York: United Nations. http://www.unodc.org/unodc/en/data-and-analysis/WDR-2005.html

UNODC (2006). *World Drug Report 2006. Volume 1: Analysis.* Vienna: United Nations Office on Drugs and Crime.

UNODC (2007). *World Drug Report 2007. Volume 1: Analysis.* Vienna: United Nations Office on Drugs and Crime.

UNODC (2008). *World Drug Report 2008.* New York: United Nations. http://www.unodc.org/unodc/en/data-and-analysis/WDR-2008.html

UNODC and Ministry of Social Justice and Empowerment, Government of India. (2004). *The Extent, Pattern and Trends of Drug Abuse in India: National Survey.* New Delhi: Ministry of Social Justice and Empowerment, Government of India and United Nations Office on Drugs and Crime Regional Office for South Asia.

Urbanosk, K.A., Strike C.J. & Rush, B. (2005). Individuals seeking treatment for cannabis-related problems in Ontario: Demographic and treatment profile. *European Addiction Research*, 11: 115–123.

US House of Representatives, United States General Accounting Office (2002). *Marijuana, Early Experiences with Four States' Laws That Allow Use for Medical Purposes.* Wachington D.C.: United States General Accounting Office.

Van der Heijden, T. (2007). *Sizing the Dutch Cannabis Market*. Unpublished presentation, EMCDDA.

Van Dijk, J. (1998). The narrow margins of the Dutch drug policy: A cost-benefit analysis. *European Journal on Criminal Policy and Research*, 6: 369–94.

Van het Loo, M., Hoorens, S., van't Hof, C. & Kahan, J. (2003). *Cannabis Policy*. Santa Monica: RAND Europe.

Van Os, J., Bak, M., Hanssen, M., Bijl, R.V., de Graaf, R. & Verdoux, H. (2002). Cannabis use and psychosis: a longitudinal population-based study. *American Journal of Epidemiology*, 156: 319–27.

Van Vliet, H.J. (1990). Separation of drug markets and the normalization of drug problems in the Netherlands: An example for other nations? *Journal of Drug Issues*, 20: 463–71.

Wachtel, S.R., ElSohly, M.A., Ross, S.A., Ambre, J. & de Wit, H. (2002). Comparison of the subjective effects of Delta(9)-tetrahydrocannabinol and marijuana in humans. *Psychopharmacology*, 161: 331–9.

Wagner, F.A. & Anthony, J.C. (2002). Into the world of illegal drug use: Exposure opportunity and other mechanisms linking the use of alcohol, tobacco, marijuana, and cocaine. *American Journal of Epidemiology*, 155: 918–25.

Warburton, C. (1932). *The Economic Results of Prohibition*. New York: Columbia University Press.

Warburton, H., May, T. & Hough, M. (2005). Looking the other way: The impact of reclassifying cannabis on police warnings, arrests and informal action in England and Wales. *British Journal of Criminology*, 45: 113–28.

Weatherburn, D. & Jones, C. (2001). *Does Prohibition Deter Cannabis Use?* Crime Bulletin Number 58, Bureau of Crime Statistics and Research. Sydney: NSW Attorney General's Department. http://www.lawlink.nsw.gov.au/lawlink/bocsar/ll_bocsar.nsf/vwFiles/cjb58.pdf/$file/cjb58.pdf

Weitzer, R. & Tuch, S. (1999). Race, class, and perceptions of discrimination by the police. *Crime & Delinquency*, 45: 494–507.

West, J. (2000) Prostitution: collectives and the politics of regulation. *Gender, Work & Organization* 7(2): 106–119.

WHO (2005). *Framework Convention on Tobacco Control*. Geneva: World Health Organization. http://www.who.int/tobacco/framework/WHO_FCTC_english.pdf

WHO Programme on Substance Abuse (1997). *Cannabis: A Health Perspective and Research Agenda*. Geneva: Division of Mental Health and Prevention of Substance Abuse, World Health Organization. Available at: http://whqlibdoc.who.int/hq/1997/WHO_MSA_PSA_97.4.pdf

Wikipedia (2008a). Bhang. (Sighted 20 August 2008). http://en.wikipedia.org/wiki/bhang

Wikipedia (2008b). Cooking with cannabis. (sighted 17 August, 2008) http://en.wikipedia.org/wiki/Cooking_with_cannabis

Wikipedia (2009). Cannabis Social Club. (sighted 29 March, 2009) http://en.wikipedia.org/wiki/Cannabis_Social_Club

Wikitravel (2008). India. (Sighted 20 August 2008). http://wikitravel.org/en/india

Wilkins, C., Casswell, S., Bhatta, K. & Pledger, M. (2002). *Drug Use in New Zealand: National Surveys Comparison 1998 and 2001*. Auckland: Alcohol and Public Health Research Unit, University of Auckland.

Wilkins, C., Reilly, J., Pledger M. & Casswell S. (2005). Estimating the dollar value of the illicit market for cannabis in New Zealand. *Drug and Alcohol Review*, 24: 227–34.

Williams, J. (2004). The effects of price and policy on marijuana use: what can be learned from the Australian experience? *Health Economics*, 13: 123–37.

Williams, J. & Mahmoudi, P. (2004) Economic relationship between alcohol and cannabis revisited. *Economic Record* 80: 36–48.

Wilson, W., Mathew, R., Turkington, T., Hawk, T., Coleman, R.E. & Provenzale, J. (2000). Brain morphological changes and early marijuana use: A magnetic resonance and positron emission tomography study. *Journal of Addictive Diseases*, 19: 1–22.

Winters, K.C. & Lee, C.Y.S. (2008). Likelihood of developing an alcohol and cannabis use disorder during youth: Association with recent use and age. *Drug and Alcohol Dependence*, 92(1–3): 239–47.

Yamaguchi, K. & Kandel, D.B. (1984). Patterns of drug use from adolescence to young adulthood: III. Predictors of progression. *American Journal of Public Health*, 74: 673–81.

Yücel, M., Solowij, N., Respondek, C., Whittle, S., Fornito, A., Pantelis, C., *et al.* (2008). Regional brain abnormalities associated with long-term heavy cannabis use. *Archives of General Psychiatry*, 65: 694–701.

Zabransky, T. (2004). Czech drug laws as an arena of the drug policy battle. *Journal of Drug Issues*, 34: 661–85.

Zabransky, T., Mravčik, V., Gajdošikova, H. & Miovsky, M. (2001). *PAD: Impact Analysis Project of New Drugs Legislation (Summary Final Report)*. Prague: Office of the Czech Governmment, Secretariat of the National Drug Commission. http://www.ak-ps.cz/client/files/PAD_en.pdf

Zaluar, A. (n.d.) *Violence Related to Illegal Drugs, 'Easy Money' and Justice in Brazil: 1980–1995*. Discussion paper No. 35. Paris: UNESCO, Management of Social Transformations (MOST) Programme. http://www.unesco.org/most/zaluar.htm [accessed December 26, 2008]

Zammit, S., Allebeck, P., Andréasson, S., Lundberg, I. & Lewis, G. (2002). Self reported cannabis use as a risk factor for schizophrenia in Swedish conscripts of 1969: Historical cohort study. *BMJ*, 325: 1199–201.

Zammit, S., Spurlock, G., Williams, H., Norton, N., Williams, N., O'Donovan, M.C., *et al.* (2007). Genotype effects of CHRNA7, CNR1 and COMT in schizophrenia: interactions with tobacco and cannabis use. *British Journal of Psychiatry*, 191: 402–07.

Zeese, K.B. (1999). History of medical marijuana policy in US. *International Journal of Drug Policy*, 10: 319–28.

Zhang, Z.F., Morgenstern, H., Spitz, M.R., Tashkin, D.P., Yu, G.P., Marshall, J.R., *et al.* (1999). Marijuana use and increased risk of squamous cell carcinoma of the head and neck. *Cancer Epidemiology, Biomarkers and Prevention*, 8: 1071–8.

Zimmer, L. & Morgan, J.P. (1997). *Marijuana Myths, Marijuana Facts: A Review of the Scientific Evidence*. New York: The Lindesmith Center.

Zuckerman, B., Frank, D.A., Hingson, R., Amaro, H., Levenson, S.M., Kayne, H., *et al.* (1989). Effects of maternal marijuana and cocaine use on fetal growth. *New England Journal of Medicine*, 320: 762–8.

About the authors and The Beckley Foundation

Robin Room is a sociologist who is a Professor at the School of Population Health, University of Melbourne, and the director of the AER Centre for Alcohol Policy Research at Turning Point Alcohol & Drug Centre, Fitzroy, Victoria, Australia. He is also a professor at and was the founding director of the Centre for Social Research on Alcohol and Drugs at Stockholm University. He had previously directed research at the Addiction Research Foundation of Ontario (1991–1998) and the Alcohol Research Group in Berkeley, California (1977–1991). Room has studied effects of alcohol, drug, and gambling policies. He is a co-author of a number of books on alcohol and drug issues, including *Young Men and Drugs* (NIDA, 1975), *Alcohol in Developing Societies* (Finnish Foundation for Alcohol Studies, 2002), and *Alcohol – No Ordinary Commodity* (Oxford UP, 2003). His research interests include historical, cultural, and social epidemiological studies of alcohol and other drugs, including comparative research across psychoactive substances.

Benedikt Fischer is Professor in the Faculty of Health Sciences and the School of Criminology, as well as Interim Director of the Centre for Applied Research in Addictions and Mental Health (CARMHA), at Simon Fraser University, Vancouver, Canada, where he also currently holds a CIHR/PHAC Research Chair in Applied Public Health and is a MSFHR Senior Scholar Career Investigator. He is furthermore an Affiliate Scientist with the BC Centre for Disease Control (BCCDC) and a Senior Scientist with the Centre for Addiction and Mental Health (CAMH) in Toronto; he co-headed the Research Section on 'Public Health and Regulatory Policies' at CAMH until his move to British Columbia in 2006. Dr. Fischer is a member of the Institute Advisory Board of the Canadian Institutes of Health Research's (CIHR) Institute for Neurosciences, Mental Health and Addiction (INHMA), as well as a member of the Science Advisory Board of the Mental Health Commission of Canada. In the course of his research, which focuses primarily on substance use, infectious disease, criminal justice and public health, Dr. Fischer has authored numerous studies on drug policy at the national and international level. In the late 1990s, he led the writing of a study by a pan-Canadian working group for options for cannabis control reform in Canada. He currently leads a CIHR-funded study developing a public health framework and interventions for cannabis use in Canada.

Wayne Hall is Professor of Public Health Policy in the School of Population Health, University of Queensland. He was formerly Director of the Office of Public Policy and Ethics at the Institute for Molecular Bioscience, UQ (2001–2005) and Director of the National Drug and Alcohol Research Centre at UNSW (1994–2001). With Rosalie Pacula, he is the author of *Cannabis Use and Dependence: Public Health and Public Policy* (Cambridge UP, 2003). He has advised the WHO on: the health effects of cannabis use; the effectiveness of drug substitution treatment; the scientific quality of the Swiss heroin trials; the contribution of illicit drug use to the global burden of disease; and the ethical implications of genetic and neuroscience research on addiction. He is currently researching: the policy and ethical implications of research on the genetics and neurobiology of nicotine dependence, biological interventions that purport to extend human life expectancy, and the regulation of pharmaceutical drugs.

Simon Lenton is a Professor and Deputy Director at the National Drug Research Institute, Perth, Western Australia, and he works as a Clinical Psychologist in private practice. He has published more than 30 scientific articles, book chapters, and reports on cannabis, health and the law and presented on the topic at numerous national and international conferences. He is first author of *Cannabis Possession, Use and Supply*, a monograph published in 2000. Lenton was a former member of the Ministerial Working Party on Drug Law Reform which advised the Western Australian Government on the design and implementation of the Cannabis Infringement Notice scheme which came into effect in March 2004. He is currently heading a large pre-post evaluation of that scheme. Lenton's research interests include illicit drug use and harm reduction, impact of legislative options for cannabis, and drink and drug driving.

Peter Reuter is an economist and public policy researcher who is a Professor in the School of Public Policy and in the Department of Criminology at the University of Maryland. He is the Director of the Program on the Economics of Crime and Justice Policy at the University and also Senior Economist at RAND. Reuter founded and directed RAND's mutlidisciplinary Drug Policy Research Center from 1989–1993. His early research focused on the organization of illegal markets and resulted in the publication of *Disorganized Crime: The Economics of the Visible Hand* (MIT Press, 1983). Since 1985 most of his research has dealt with alternative approaches to controlling drug problems, both in the United States and Western Europe. His other books are (with Robert MacCoun) *Drug War Heresies: Learning from Other Places, Times and*

Vices (Cambridge UP, 2001) and (with Edwin Truman) *Chasing Dirty Money: The Fight Against Money Laundering* (Institute for International Economics, 2004) and (with Letizia Paoli and Victoria Greenfield) *The World Heroin Market: Can Supply be Cut?* (Oxford). In 2007 he was elected the first president of the International Society for the Study of Drug Policy.

Amanda Feilding, founder and director of The Beckley Foundation, has long advocated an evidence-based approach to drug policy that seeks to minimize the harms associated with drug use. Towards this end she has hosted seven influential seminars on International Drug Policy issues, entitled '*Society and Drugs: A Rational Perspective*'. These meetings bring together leading academics, experts and policy-makers from around the world, and have helped not only to broaden the debate, but also initiated such innovations as the 2007 call for a UK drug-classification system based on a scientifically-evaluated scale of harms. In 2006, her awareness of the lack of attention paid to cannabis in international drug policy discussions led her to convene the Global Cannabis Commission Report.

The Beckley Foundation is an ECOSOC-accredited NGO, whose Drug Policy Programme was set up to develop a scientifically-evaluated evidence base on which drug policy could be reliably based. It aims to cast light on the current dilemmas facing policy-makers within governments and international agencies, and to work with them in order to promote objective and open debate on the effectiveness, direction, and content of future drug policies.

The Foundation has produced over 30 academic reports, proceedings documents and briefing papers on key policy questions and recent policy initiatives. It has founded two sister organizations, both now independent: the *International Society for the Study of Drug Policy* (ISSDP) and the *International Drug Policy Consortium* (IDPC).

Underlying the Beckley's drug policy programme are a number of observations:

- That the current global drug control mechanism (as enshrined in the three United Nations Conventions of 1961, 1971 and 1988), is not achieving the core objective of significantly reducing the scale of the market for controlled substances, such as heroin, cocaine, methamphetamine, and cannabis.

- That the negative side-effects of the implementation of this system may themselves be creating significant social problems.

- That reducing the harm faced by the many individuals who use drugs, including the risk of infections, such as Hepatitis C and HIV/AIDS, does not hold a sufficiently high priority in international policies and programmes.

- That there is a growing body of evidence regarding which policies and activities are (and are not) effective in reducing drug use and associated health and social problems, and that this evidence is not sufficiently taken into account in current policy discussions, which continue to be dominated by ideological considerations.

- That the current dilemmas in international drug policy can only be resolved through an honest review of progress so far, a better understanding of the complex factors that create widespread drug use, and a commitment to pursue policies that are effective.

- That analysis of future policy options is unlikely to produce a clear, single 'correct' policy – what may be appropriate in one setting or culture may be less so in another. In addition, there are likely to be trade-offs between policy objectives (e.g. to reduce overall drug use or to reduce drug-related crime) that may be viewed differently in different countries.

- That future policy should be grounded on a scientifically based scale of harm for all social drugs, both legal and illegal. This should involve a continuous review of scientific and sociological evidence of their biological harms, toxicity, mortality, and dependency; of their relation to violent behaviour; of their relation to crime; of their costs to the health services; of their general impact on the community; and of the total economic impact of the use of each individual drug on society.

The Beckley Foundation also runs a parallel Scientific Programme which promotes the scientific investigation of consciousness and its changing states from a multidisciplinary perspective. Working in collaboration with leading scientists and institutions around the world it initiates and directs research into the neurophysiology underlying the full range of conscious states. It is particularly interested in scientific research that has practical implications for improving health and well-being, and which also provides the scientific evidence upon which better informed policy decisions can be based.

Index